ICP-IAN
100 Questions in
Neurological Practice

Office Neurology, Neuro Muscular and Functional Neurology

VIDEO CONTENTS

SECTION 3: FUNCTIONAL NEUROLOGY

Video 1: Video shows how during the Romberg test, the boy shows functional imbalance. He tends to lose balance to either side when performing the Romberg test.

Video 2: When his attention is diverted by asking him to do dysdiadochokinesis test with feet close and eyes open and closed as in the Romberg's he no longer loses balance.

Video 3: La belle indifference observed in a lady with tremor of the left side of her face for the past six months. She does not appear particularly concerned by it and is quite cheerful when describing it.

Video 4: This is called the whack-a-mole sign. When the tremor is prevented in one area, for example in the thumb, it happens in the hands, or later in the feet.

Video 5: This sign is called distractibility. Observe the tremor in the left hand and note how it reduces and even stops when he is asked to do finger tapping with the right hand.

Video 6: This is suggestibility. The apparent dystonia of the lip and jaw muscles as well as the eyes, is induced by suggestion. By placing a tuning fork and informing the patient that the application of the tuning fork might very likely induce the abnormal movement, it does indeed occur.

Video 7: This is called astasia abasia. Here is a patient who is complaining of imbalance while walking. However, upon observing his gait, he demonstrates exquisite balance. He sways wildly from side to side yet still maintains his balance even on one foot and does not fall.

Video 8: This boy demonstrates intermittent loss of balance toward the right side initially when he is walking. Later, when he turns around, he still loses balance, but now to the left side.

Video 9: This girl demonstrates a type of functional gait, in which she drags the leg like a stick.

Video 10: This is another example of dragging the leg like a stick.

Video 11: This lady with functional imbalance of gait shows a peculiar hiccup-like movement of the upper body when standing and walking but when lying in bed this stops and she shows a slower flexion extension at the ankles.

Video 12: This is another example of a functional gait, where the patient for every few steps ahead, suddenly takes backward steps without losing balance and this cycle continues.

Video 13: Another example of astasia abasia. A wildly swaying gait without losing balance. She also demonstrates giving way at the knees without falling.

Video 14: This girl demonstrates functional falls in which she surveys the terrain and make sure that she will not get hurt before she falls. There is no loss of consciousness and her gait is quite normal before she falls.

Video 15: The tremor in the left side of the face stops when she is asked to show her teeth. In addition there is peculiar crossed tremor with an irregular tremor in the right hand.

Video 16: A girl with functional seizures who resists eye opening and shows Bell's phenomenon when we tried to force open her eyes. She seems to have to do a lot of exertion and then the attack stops suddenly without any post-ictal confusion.

Video 17: Functional seizures induced by suggestion in a boy. He demonstrates irregular movements of both legs which are not typical tonic clonic jerking as we see in epilepsy. Also he is fully conscious and shows his tongue when asked to.

Video 18: Another boy with functional seizures induced by suggestion by using a tuning fork for suggestion. Before applying the tuning fork, we tell the patient that often this machine can induce an attack. We must make sure that this induced attack is the same as his usual attacks. Also note how it stops suddenly as soon as we tell him to stop.

Video 19: Spasm of convergence in a girl whose complaining of blurring of vision.

Video 20: Peculiar stuttering of voice when the person tries to speak and many makes an effort to speak his whole body starts shaking and trembling.

Video 21: This is functional dysphonia in which the person suddenly starts whispering. He tries to speak and enunciate the words but whispers. His cough is quite normal unlike what would happen with a laryngeal disorder.

Please scan the QR code to access the videos

ICP-IAN
100 Questions in
Neurological Practice

Office Neurology, Neuro Muscular and Functional Neurology

Editors

PK Maheshwari
MD DM(Neurology) MAMS FFIACM FRCP(Edinburgh) FIAN FICP
Professor and Head
Department of Neurology
Erstwhile Director–Professor and Head
PG Department of Medicine
Sarojini Naidu Medical College
Agra, Uttar Pradesh, India
President, Agra Academy of Neurology
Honorary Secretary, Agra Branch, Association of Physician of India

Sangeeta Ravat
MD(General Medicine) DM(Neurology) FIAN
Professor
Department of Neurology
Chief Epileptologist, Comprehensive Epilepsy Care Center
Dean, Seth GS Medical College and KEM Hospital
Fellow, Pediatric Neurology Department at Royal Children's Hospital, Melbourne
President, Mumbai Chapter of Indian Epilepsy Association (SAMMAN)
President Indian Academy of Neurology

Forewords

Jyotirmoy Pal **Bhim Singhal** **RK Singal** **Devika Nag**
Milind Nadkar **Man Mohan Mehndiratta** **BB Thakur** **Nirmal Surya**

JAYPEE BROTHERS MEDICAL PUBLISHERS
The Health Sciences Publisher
New Delhi | London

Jaypee Brothers Medical Publishers (P) Ltd

Headquarters
EMCA House
23/23-B, Ansari Road, Daryaganj
New Delhi 110 002, India
Landline: +91-11-23272143, +91-11-23272703
+91-11-23282021, +91-11-23245672
E-mail: jaypee@jaypeebrothers.com

Corporate Office
Jaypee Brothers Medical Publishers (P) Ltd.
4838/24, Ansari Road, Daryaganj
New Delhi 110 002, India
Phone: +91-11-43574357
Fax: +91-11-43574314
E-mail: jaypee@jaypeebrothers.com

Overseas Office
JP Medical Ltd.
83, Victoria Street, London
SW1H 0HW (UK)
Phone: +44-20 3170 8910
Fax: +44(0)20 3008 6180
E-mail: info@jpmedpub.com

Website: www.jaypeebrothers.com
Website: www.jaypeedigital.com

Inquiries for bulk sales may be solicited at: jaypee@jaypeebrothers.com

ICP-IAN 100 Questions in Neurological Practice 3 / PK Maheshwari, Sangeeta Ravat

First Edition: **2025**

ISBN: 978-93-6616-279-9

Printed at: Samrat Offset Pvt. Ltd.

Advisory Board

Contributors

Section Editors

Section 1: Office Neurology

Lakshmi Narasimhan Ranganathan MD(Medicine) DNB(Medicine) DM(Neurology) DrNB(Neurology) PhD(Neurology) FRCP(Glasgow) FRCP(London) FAAN FEBN FIAN FACP MNAMS
Professor and Head
Department of Neurology
Sri Ramachandra Medical College
Chennai, Tamil Nadu, India
President Elect – Indian Academy of Neurology

Biman Kanti Ray MD(Medicine) DNB(Medicine) DM(Neurology)
Professor
Department of Neurology
Bangur Institute of Neurosciences
Institute of Postgraduate Medical Education and Research
Kolkata, West Bengal, India

Section 2: Neuro Muscular

Satish Khadilkar MD DM DNBE FIAN FICP FAMS FRCP
Dean and Professor and Head
Department of Neurology
Bombay Hospital Institute of Medical Sciences
Mumbai, Maharashtra, India
Past President – Indian Academy of Neurology

Achal Kumar Srivastava MD DM(Neurology) FRCP(London) FAAN FANA FNASc FIAN FAMS FICP
Professor
Department of Neurology
All India Institute of Medical Sciences
New Delhi, India
Treasurer Indian Academy of Neurology
Secretary Delhi Neurological Association
Secretory Nerve Muscle Society

Section 3: Functional Neurology

Sudhir Kothari MD(Medicine) DM(Neurology) FRCP (London) FIAN
Head
Department of Neurology
Poona Hospital and Research Centre
Managing Trustee, FINE (Forum for Indian Neurology Education)
Pune, Maharashtra, India

Hrishikesh Kumar MD DM PDF
Head
Department of Neurology
Vice Chairman
Institute of Neurosciences
Kolkata, West Bengal, India

Associate Editors

Shrivarthan R MD(Medicine) DM(Neurology) DrNB(Neurology) MRCP(SCE) FEBN
Consultant Neurologist
MGM Healthcare
Chennai, Tamil Nadu, India

Ashok Kumar MD DM
Professor and Head
Department of Neurology
Indira Gandhi Institute of Medical Sciences
Patna, Bihar, India

Ayush Agarwal MD DM DNB MNAMS Associate FAMS
Assistant Professor
Department of Neurology
All India Institute of Medical Sciences
New Delhi, India

Jacky Ganguly MD DM PDF
Consultant Neurologist
Institute of Neurosciences
Kolkata, West Bengal, India

Eish Kumar Dalla MD(Psychiatry)
Consultant Psychiatrist
JLN District Hospital
Rudrapur, Uttarakhand, India

Navneet Agrawal MD(Medicine) DM(Neurology)
Assistant Professor
Department of Neurology
Sarojini Naidu Medical College
Agra, Uttar Pradesh, India

Rajesh Verma MD(Medicine) DM(Neurology) DNB(Neurology)
Professor
Department of Neurology
King George's Medical University
Lucknow, Uttar Pradesh, India

Abhijeet Gadhave MD
Senior Resident
Department of Neurology
Bombay Hospital Institute of Medical Sciences
Mumbai, Maharashtra, India

Soaham Desai MD DM(Neurology)
Senior Consultant Neurologist
Shree Krishna Hospital
Professor and Head
Department of Neurology
Pramukhswami Medical College
Bhaikaka University
Anand, Gujarat, India

Parthvi Ravat MD DrNB(Neurology) FRACP Trainee
Fellow in Epilepsy
Flinders Medical Centre
Adelaide, Australia

Foreword

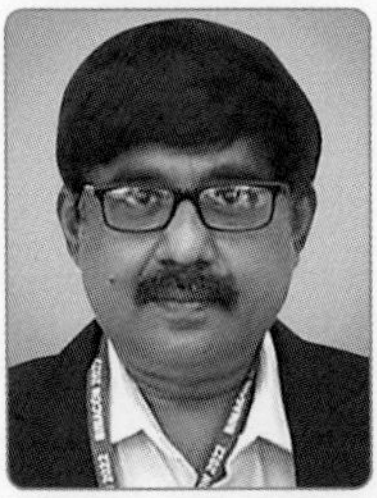

Jyotirmoy Pal MBBS MD(General Medicine) FRCP FICP FACP
WHO Fellow
Professor, Department of Medicine
College of Medicine and Sagore Dutta Hospital
Kolkata, West Bengal, India
Past Dean, Indian College of Physicians (ICP)
Chairman, Scientific Committee, Association of Physicians of India
President-Elect, Association of Physicians of India

In today's fast-paced medical landscape, a thorough understanding of neurology—blending foundational knowledge with practical application—is essential. The *"ICP-IAN 100 Questions in Neurological Practice 3"* first edition provides just that, offering an in-depth exploration of Office Neurology, Neuromuscular, and Functional Neurology.

What sets this book apart is its ability to bridge the gap between theoretical knowledge and real-world practice. The clarity of thought, meticulous organization, and practical focus presented by chief editors Drs *PK Maheshwari* and *Sangeeta Ravat* make this a quintessential guide for all neurologists and physicians.

Jyotirmoy Pal

Foreword

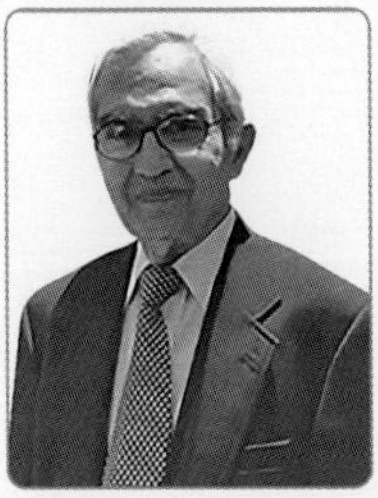

Bhim Singhal MD DSc FRCP(London, Edinburgh) FAMS
Director
Department of Neurology
Bombay Hospital and Medical Research Centre
Mumbai, Maharashtra, India

Few books manage to achieve the perfect balance of being comprehensive and accessible, but this edition of "*ICP-IAN 100 Questions in Neurological Practice 3*" does so with grace and precision. Addressing the critical areas of Office Neurology, Neuro Muscular, and Functional Neurology, it provides a roadmap for navigating the challenges of modern medical practice. Modern medicine thrives on innovation and precision, and this book embodies these principles. It provides an up-to-date and comprehensive view of the field.

Chief editors Drs *PK Maheshwari* and *Sangeeta Ravat* have demonstrated exemplary leadership and insight in curating this edition. It is a resource that will undoubtedly leave a lasting impact on its readers and the field of neurology at large.

Bhim Singhal

Foreword

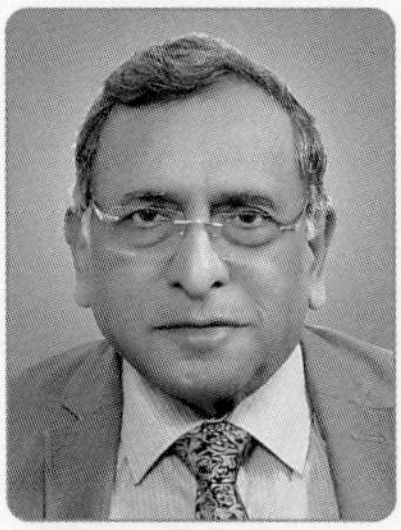

RK Singal MD(General Medicine) FICP FACP(USA) FIAMS
Dean ICP
Past President API
Principal Director and Head, Department of Internal Medicine
BLK-MAX Super Speciality Hospital
New Delhi, India

As the Dean of the Indian College of Physicians (ICP), the esteemed academic wing dedicated to the advancement of internal medicine in India, it is with great pleasure that I introduce the latest edition of *"ICP-IAN 100 Questions in Neurological Practice (Volume 3)."*

The collaboration between the ICP and the Indian Academy of Neurology (IAN) in producing this monograph underscores our commitment to interdisciplinary education and excellence in patient care. By bridging the gap between internal medicine and neurology, this publication equips internists with the knowledge to make informed decisions, ultimately enhancing patient outcomes.

Neurology often presents intricate challenges in clinical practice, requiring a nuanced understanding of various subspecialties. This edition of *"ICP-IAN 100 Questions in Neurological Practice 3"* emerges as a cornerstone for those seeking clarity and depth in neurology. Addressing key areas such as Office Neurology, Neuro Muscular, and Functional Neurology, it is both a practical guide and an academic resource. These sections of this book are thoughtfully curated to address the pressing needs of neurologists and physicians alike. I am confident that this edition will serve as a practical and academic cornerstone for its readers.

Chief editors Drs *PK Maheshwari* and *Sangeeta Ravat* have brought together a wealth of knowledge, ensuring that this edition remains relevant and engaging. Its structure allows for easy navigation and practical application, making it an invaluable resource for students and professionals alike.

I am confident that this monograph will serve as a trusted companion for both neurologists and internists, enriching their practice and fostering a deeper understanding of neurological conditions.

RK Singal

Foreword

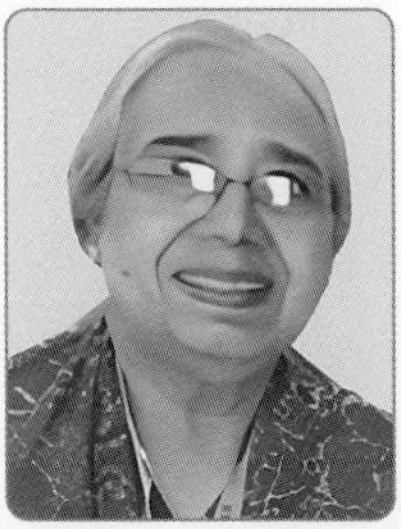

Devika Nag MD FAAN
Emeritus Professor Neurology
Former Head, Department of Neurology
KG Medical College Lucknow, Uttar Pradesh, India
Past President, Indian Academy of Neurology

The field of neurology stands at the forefront of medical innovation, with new discoveries reshaping our understanding and practice. This new edition of "*ICP-IAN 100 Questions in Neurological Practice 3*" reflects these advancements, presenting three core sections that resonate with contemporary challenges: Office Neurology, Neuro Muscular, and Functional Neurology. The seamless blending of theory and practice in this edition is remarkable.

Under the skilled guidance of chief editors Drs *PK Maheshwari* and *Sangeeta Ravat*, this book not only educates but also inspires. It is a must-have resource for anyone invested in mastering the complexities of neurology.

Devika Nag

Foreword

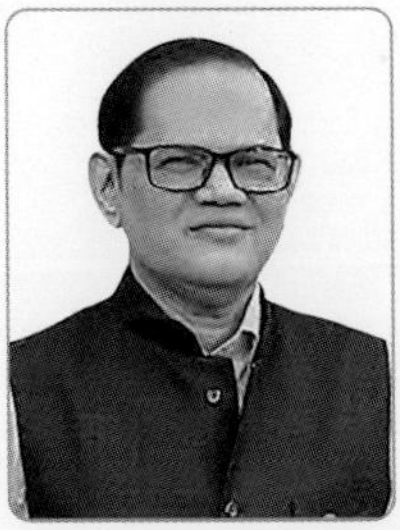

Milind Nadkar MD FICP FACP
Professor and Head
Department of Medicine and Chief of Rheumatology
Seth GS Medical College and KEM Hospital
Mumbai, Maharashtra, India
President
Association of Physicians of India (API)

This edition of "*ICP-IAN 100 Questions in Neurological Practice 3*" is a celebration of knowledge and collaboration, presenting neurology in a manner that is both profound and practical. The sections on Office Neurology, Neuro Muscular, and Functional Neurology encapsulate the diversity and depth of the field. Every edition of a book carries the promise of updated knowledge and expanded horizons, and this edition fulfils this promise.

The editorial team, led by Drs *PK Maheshwari* and *Sangeeta Ravat*, has succeeded in crafting a resource that speaks to both academic rigor and clinical relevance. Their effort ensures that this book will serve as a cornerstone for medical education and practice.

Milind Nadkar

Foreword

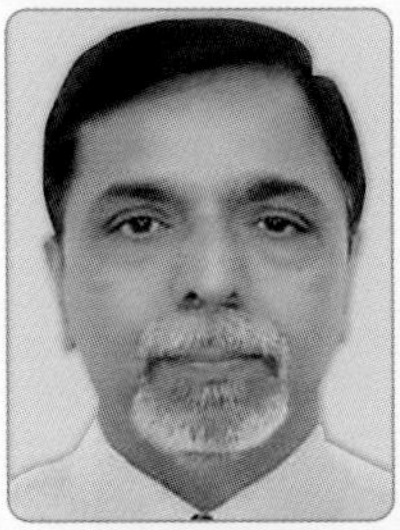

Man Mohan Mehndiratta MD DNB DM (Neurology) FAAN FANA FAMS FRCP FICP FIAN FIACM

Past-President, Indian Academy of Neurology

Emeritus Professor of National Academy of Medical Sciences (India)

Currently: Principal–Director, Department of Neurology

BLK-Max Super Speciality Hospital (Max Health Care Group),

Center for Neurosciences

New Delhi, India

Neurology has always been a subject that inspires awe and curiosity, given its complexity and relevance to the human experience. This new edition of "*ICP-IAN 100 Questions in Neurological Practice 3*" continues to build on the strengths of its predecessors, presenting a refined and contemporary perspective on Office Neurology, Neuro Muscular, and Functional Neurology.

The ability to simplify complex concepts while maintaining scientific rigor is a hallmark of this work. Through the efforts of chief editors, Drs *PK Maheshwari* and *Sangeeta Ravat*, this edition is a testament to their dedication and understanding of the needs of the modern medical community. It will undoubtedly prove to be a beacon of guidance for many.

Man Mohan Mehndiratta

Foreword

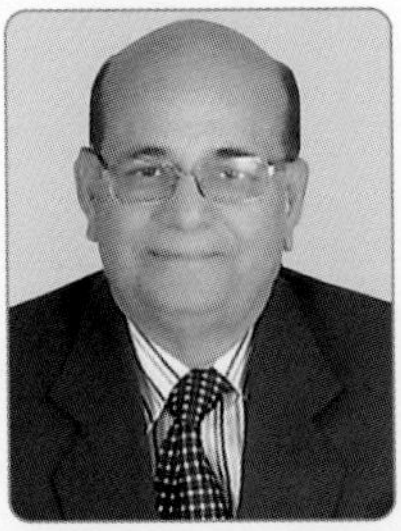

BB Thakur MD FICP FIAMS FIACM FACP FISPD
Past Dean, ICP
Past President, API
Past President, Hypertension Society of India
Retired Professor and Head, Department of Medicine
Sri Krishna Medical College and Hospital
Muzaffarpur, Bihar, India

It gives me immense pleasure and pride to write the foreword for "*ICP-IAN 100 Questions in Neurological Practice 3*".

The ever-evolving challenges in neurological practice that an internist and neurologists face in their day-to-day practice require resources beyond journals and libraries which are easily available, handy, and academically robust, relevant, and practical.

This edition of "*ICP-IAN 100 Questions in Neurological Practice 3*" has been very meticulously curated by chief editors Drs *PK Maheshwari* and *Sangeeta Ravat* who have done that job very precisely and divided it into three crucial sections—Office Neurology, Neuro Muscular, and Functional Neurology.

It is accessible format and thoughtful content ensure that it caters to seasoned practitioners and budding neurologists alike.

This work in continuity is a testament to the editorial team's vision and dedication in advancing the knowledge in the field of neurology for which I commend them profusely.

I am confident that this incredible work will meet the aspirations of the medical fraternity, which is looking for in-depth knowledge in clinical neurology.

Warm regards,

BB Thakur

Foreword

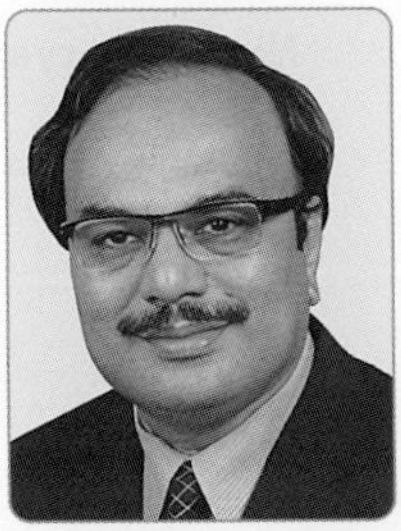

Nirmal Surya MD DNB MNAMS FIAN FAAN
President (Founder)
Indian Federation of Neurorehabilitation
President, Indian Stroke Association
Past President, Indian Academy of Neurology
Founder Trustee and Chairman, Epilepsy Foundation, India

Neurology, the intricate nexus of science and compassionate care, stands as one of the most dynamic and demanding domains in medicine, requiring unyielding commitment to learning and evolution. This edition of "*ICP-IAN 100 Questions in Neurological Practice 3*" tackles three cornerstone topics: Office Neurology, Neuro Muscular, and Functional Neurology, presenting them with precision and authority.

The first section, "Office Neurology", confronts the practical challenges of outpatient neurological care with clarity and purpose. From ubiquitous conditions like migraines, back pain, and vertigo to the nuanced presentations of early neurodegenerative diseases, this section equips primary care physicians and neurologists with the tools to navigate complexities efficiently. It emphasizes a patient-centered ethos, razor-sharp diagnostic strategies, and proactive management pathways to deliver outcomes that matter.

The second section, "Neuromuscular", unveils the complexities of conditions disrupting the vital harmony between nerves and muscles. Through incisive discussions on myopathies, motor neuron diseases, and peripheral neuropathies, this section accentuates the indispensability of advanced diagnostics and cutting-edge therapies. It underscores the transformative potential of multidisciplinary collaboration in mitigating the profound challenges posed by these conditions.

The third section, "Functional Neurology", breaks boundaries, championing an innovative approach that intertwines neurological science with holistic health. By delving into the adaptability and resilience of the nervous system, this section redefines the paradigms of care for conditions such as functional neurological disorder (FND). It epitomizes the spirit of modern neurology—innovative, patient-tailored, and relentlessly forward-thinking.

The meticulous editorial leadership of chief editors Drs *PK Maheshwari* and *Sangeeta Ravat*, alongside distinguished subsection editors Drs Lakshmi Narasimhan Ranganathan, Biman Kanti Ray, Achal Kumar Srivastava, Satish

Khadilkar, Hrishikesh Kumar, Sudhir Kothari, and the dedicated associate editors, elevates this edition into an indispensable compendium. Its seamless blend of foundational knowledge and actionable insights positions it as a definitive resource for students, practitioners, and academics alike.

This is more than a book—it is a beacon of expertise, an essential ally in the pursuit of neurological excellence, and a testament to the relentless advancement of this remarkable field.

Nirmal Surya

Preface

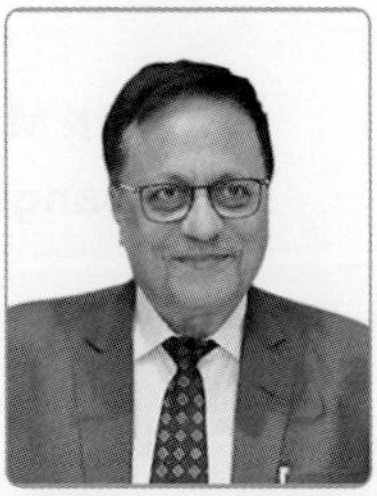

PK Maheshwari

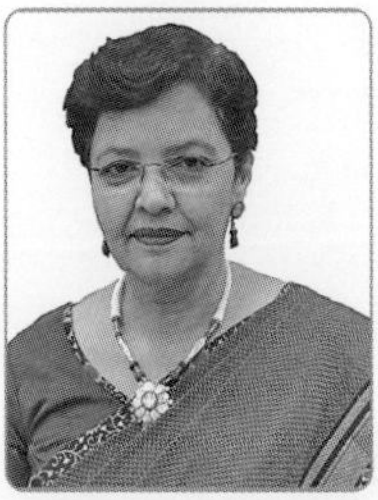

Sangeeta Ravat

The field of neurology continues to evolve rapidly, bringing both challenges and opportunities for clinicians and students. It is with great humility and dedication that we present *"ICP-IAN 100 Questions in Neurological Practice 3"*, a collaborative effort aimed at simplifying complex neurological concepts and enhancing clinical practice.

This edition marks a significant milestone in our journey. It builds upon the strengths of previous editions, incorporating the latest advancements in neurology while maintaining the concise question-and-answer format that has made this series so well regarded. Topics have been carefully curated to address the most pressing and practical issues encountered in neurological practice, ensuring relevance and applicability for a diverse readership.

The current edition includes three pivotal sections: *Office Neurology*, *Neuro Muscular*, and *Functional Neurology*. Each section has been meticulously updated by renowned experts in the field, ensuring both accuracy and clarity. This format continues to serve as an indispensable resource for practicing neurologists, postgraduate students, and general physicians seeking to enhance their understanding of neurology.

We extend our deepest gratitude to our section editors for their invaluable expertise and dedication. Our sincere thanks go to Drs **Lakshmi Narasimhan Ranganathan** and **Biman Kanti Ray** in the Office Neurology section, Drs **Satish Khadilkar** and **Achal Kumar Srivastava** in the Neuromuscular section, and Drs **Sudhir Kothari** and **Hrishikesh Kumar** in the Functional Neurology section for their outstanding contributions.

We also wish to acknowledge the remarkable efforts of our editorial team members, Shrivarthan R, Navneet Agrawal, Ashok Kumar, Rajesh Verma, Ayush Agarwal, Abhijeet Gadhave, Jacky Ganguly, Soaham Desai, Eish Kumar Dalla, and Parthvi Ravat, whose support, insight, and hard work have greatly enhanced the quality of our work.

This edition would not have been possible without the unwavering support of the Indian College of Physicians (ICP) and the Indian Academy of Neurology (IAN), whose collaboration exemplifies the spirit of academic excellence.

To all readers, we hope this book serves as a trusted guide and companion in your pursuit of neurological knowledge. We are confident that it will enrich your clinical acumen and inspire further exploration in this fascinating field of medicine.

Sincerely,

PK Maheshwari

Sangeeta Ravat

Acknowledgments

From the Convener's Desk

It is with immense pleasure that I present this book, made possible through the unwavering encouragement, support, and guidance of Dr RK Singal, Dean, Indian College of Physicians (ICP); Dr Jyotirmoy Pal, Chairman, Scientific Committee and President-Elect, Association of Physicians of India; and the office bearers of the Indian Academy of Neurology (IAN), who placed their trust in me. I extend my heartfelt thanks to ICP and IAN for their enthusiasm and invaluable support in bringing to fruition this resourceful monograph, *"ICP-IAN 100 Questions in Neurological Practice 3" (Office Neurology, Neuromuscular, and Functional Neurology)*, and for bestowing upon me the honor of serving as Editor-in-Chief. Special thanks to Dr Jyotirmoy Pal, whose contributions were pivotal in conceptualizing and creating this monograph. His meticulous discussions laid its foundation.

I am deeply grateful to the section editors and associate editors for their diligent efforts in outlining and refining the sections.

I would also like to express my gratitude to Drs Prashant Gupta, Prashant Lavania, SK Katharia, SK Majumdar, Manoj K Malav, Navneet Agrawal, and other distinguished members of the Agra Branch API, as well as members of the Agra Academy of Neurology, for their immense support throughout this journey.

I am profoundly thankful to M/s Jaypee Brothers Medical Publishers (P) Ltd, New Delhi, India, for their exceptional efforts in ensuring that this work reaches readers. My sincere thanks go to Shri Jitendar P Vij (Group Chairman) and his team, including Mr Ankit Vij (Managing Director), Mr Sabyasachi Hazra (Associate Director, Publishing and Digital Sales), Mr Priyansh Saxena (Development Editor) and the entire production team, for their steadfast support.

On a personal note, I am deeply appreciative of my beloved wife, Neetu Maheshwari, for her unconditional love and moral support. My heartfelt thanks also go to Dr Kopal, Dr Eish, Arpita, and Sambhav for their encouragement and assistance.

Finally, I extend my gratitude to my undergraduate and postgraduate students, as well as my patients, for their invaluable contributions and inspiration.

PK Maheshwari
Sangeeta Ravat

Contents

PLATE 1

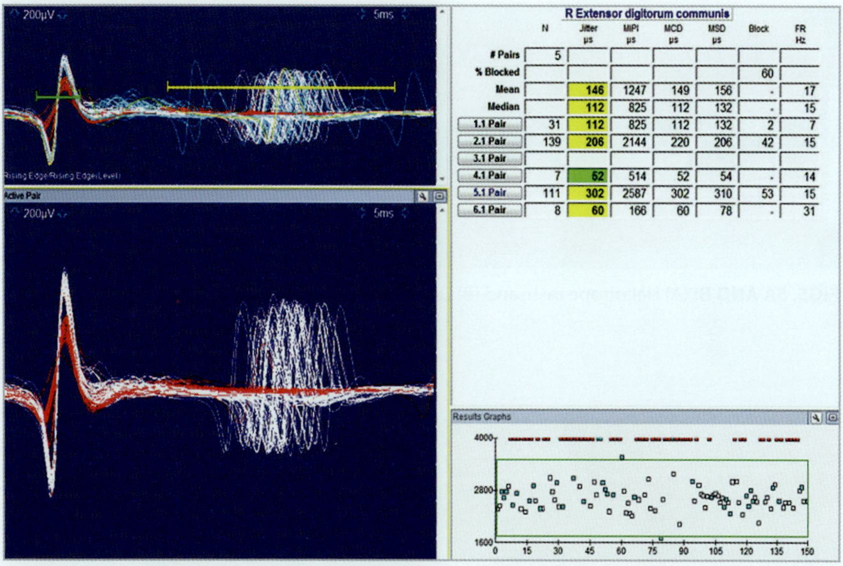

FIG. 2: Single-fiber electromyography (SFEMG) showing increased jitter in myasthenia gravis (MG). ***(Section 2)***

Courtesy: Department of Electroneuromyography, Bombay Hospital, Mumbai.

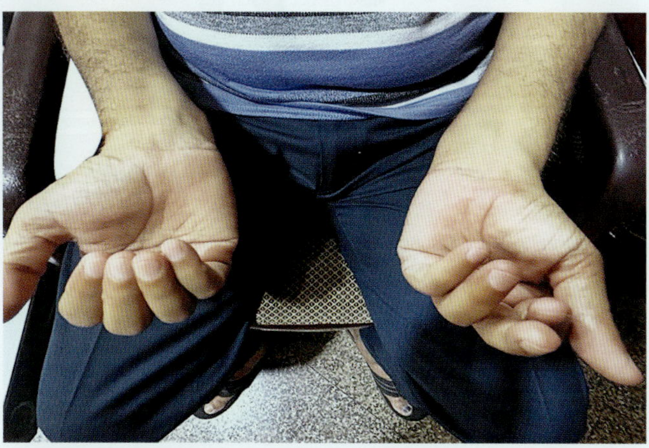

FIG. 4: On attempting to make a fist, the patient cannot fully close the hand due to finger flexor weakness in inclusion body myositis. ***(Section 2)***

PLATE 2

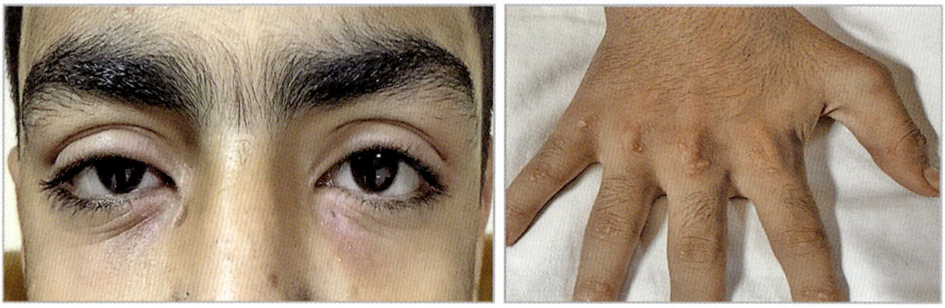

FIGS. 5A AND B: (A) Heliotrope rash; and (B) Gottron papules. ***(Section 2)***

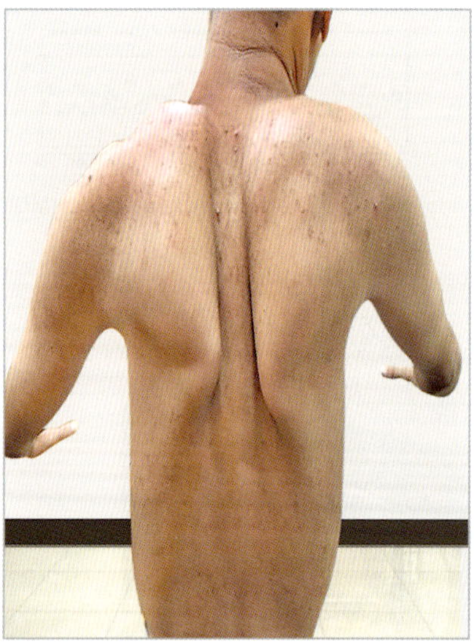

FIG. 6: Scapular winging in calpainopathy. ***(Section 2)***

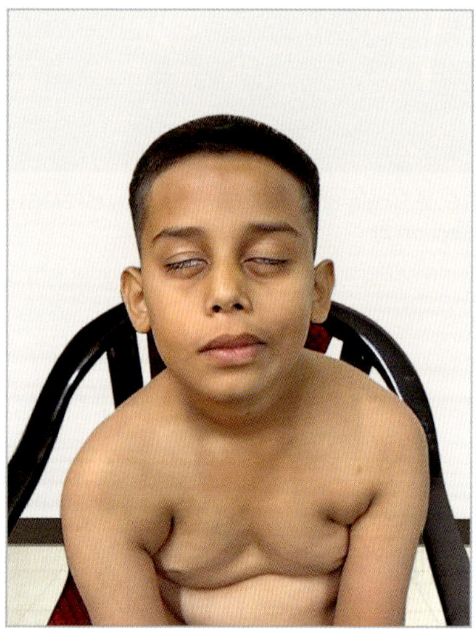

FIG. 7: Early facial involvement is seen in facioscapulohumeral muscular dystrophy (FSHD). ***(Section 2)***

PLATE 3

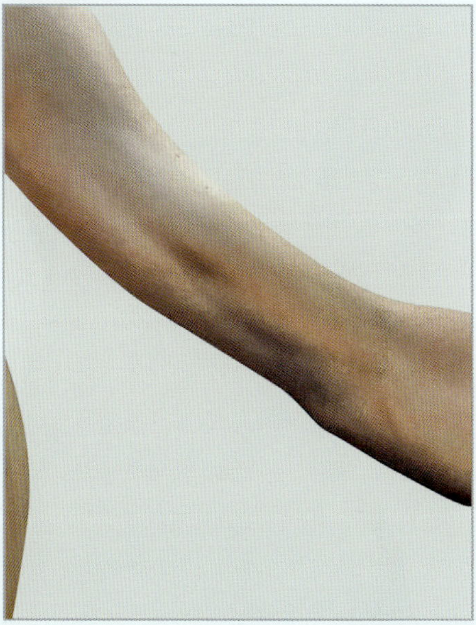

FIG. 8: Biceps lump in dysferlinopathy. ***(Section 2)***

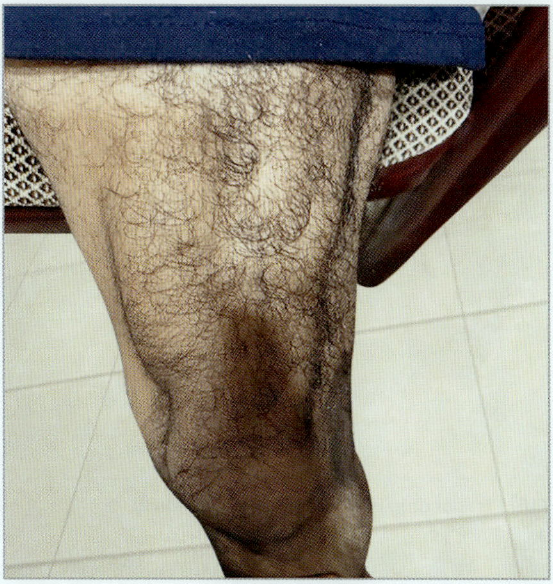

FIG. 9: Diamond on quadriceps in dysferlinopathy. ***(Section 2)***

PLATE 4

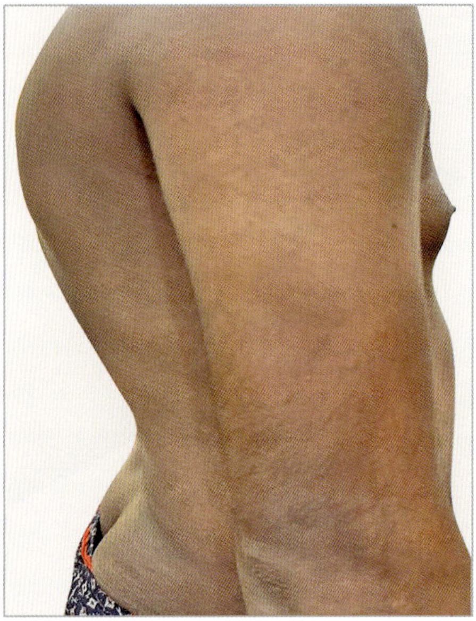

FIG. 10: Exaggerated lumbar lordosis in a patient of calpainopathy. ***(Section 2)***

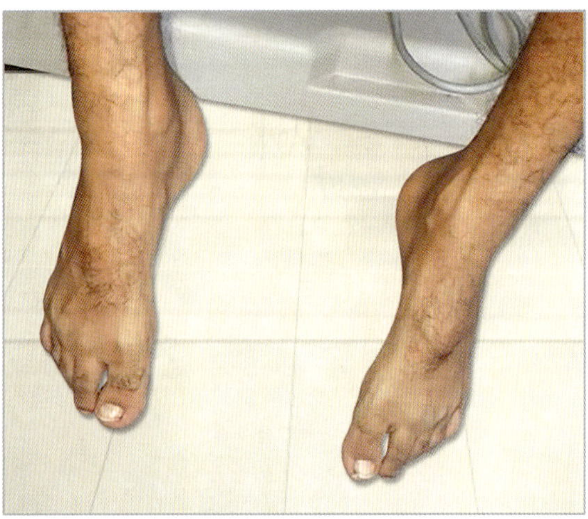

FIG. 11: Foot drop in GNE myopathy. ***(Section 2)***

PLATE 5

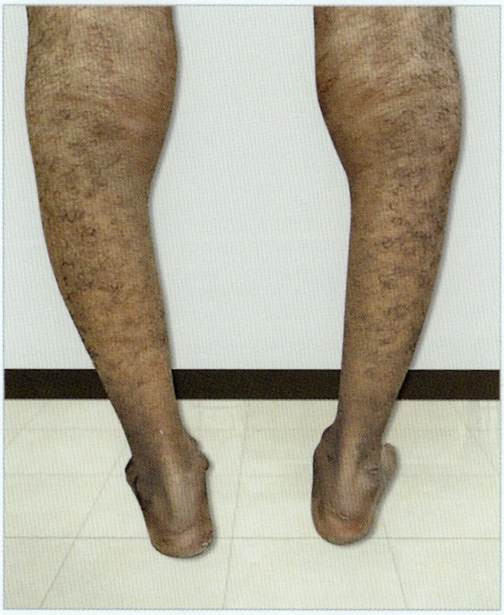

FIG. 12: Calf atrophy in dysferlinopathy. ***(Section 2)***

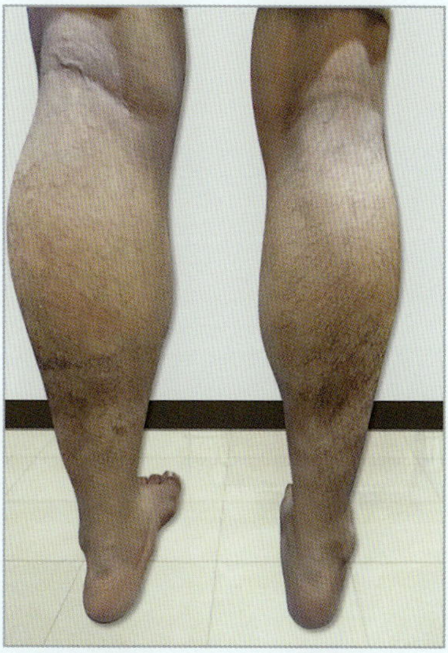

FIG. 13: Calf hypertrophy in Duchenne muscular dystrophy. ***(Section 2)***

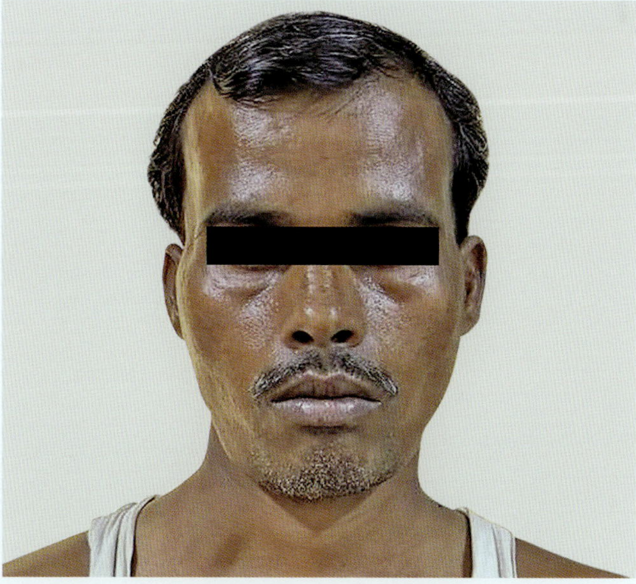

FIG. 14: Hatchet facies, frontal balding, and wasting of the temporalis muscles in myotonic muscular dystrophy. ***(Section 2)***

SECTION 1

Office Neurology

Section Editors: Lakshmi Narasimhan Ranganathan, Biman Kanti Ray

Associate Editors: Shrivarthan R, Navneet Agrawal, Ashok Kumar, Rajesh Verma

Q1. How and when to start medications for dementia?

Ans. Dementia is defined as an acquired disorder characterized by a progressive decline in cognition that affects at least one or more of the six defined cognitive domains (language, learning and memory, executive function, perceptual-motor function, complex attention, and social cognition). Alzheimer's disease (AD) is the most common cause of dementia and most medications for dementia have been predominantly studied in patients with AD. The two major group of drugs for dementia include central cholinesterase inhibitors (ChEIs) which increase the levels of cerebral acetylcholine (donepezil, rivastigmine, and galantamine) and a non-competitive NMDA receptor antagonist (memantine). Studies have shown that these agents delay disease progression, enhance cognitive functions and improve activities of daily living. At present the recommendation is to offer medications to all patients with dementia at the point of initial diagnosis **(Flowchart 1)**. Medical therapy of dementia not only includes administration of the dementia drugs but also addresses the coexistent neuropsychiatric issues and risk factor control **(Flowchart 2)**. Choosing the right agent depends on the clinical profile of the patient (disease severity), pharmacological properties of the agent and the adverse effect profile **(Table 1)**. The EFNS-ENS/EAN guideline published in 2015 favors the combination of memantine with ChEI over monotherapy in patients with moderate-to-severe dementia.

Currently 2 Food and Drug Administration (FDA)-approved amyloid targeted monoclonal antibodies are available (lecanemab and donanemab) and their use is recommended in patients with mild disease (MMSE >22, MoCA >17 or CDR 0.5 to 1) with documented amyloid pathology (amyloid PET scan or lumbar puncture).[1-3]

TABLE 1: Anti-dementia drugs, their dosing and application.

Agent	Dosing	Adverse effect	Clinical application
Donepezil	5–10 mg once daily oral medication	• Gastritis, diarrhea, and GI dysfunction • Galantamine and rivastigmine to be avoided in the setting of renal/liver disease	Mild-to-moderate AD
Galantamine	• 4 mg twice daily to 12 mg twice daily oral medication (immediate release) • 8 mg once daily to 24 mg once daily oral medication (extended release)		
Rivastigmine	• 1.5 mg twice daily to 6 mg twice daily oral medication • Transdermal patch • 4.6 mg/24 h • 9.5 mg/24 h • 13.3 mg/24 h		
Memantine	• 5 mg once daily to 10 mg twice daily oral medication (immediate release) • 7 mg once daily to 28 mg once daily oral medication (extended release)	Confusion, dizziness, drowsiness, and headache	Moderate-to-severe AD

Classification of dementia:
Mild: MMSE 19–26; MoCA 12–16; CDR 1
Moderate: MMSE 10–18; MoCA 4–11; CDR 2
Severe: MMSE <10; MoCA <4; CDR 3
(AD: Alzheimer's disease; CDR: clinical dementia rating score; MMSE: mini-mental scale examination, MoCA: Montreal cognitive assessment)

Step 1
Baseline clinical, laboratory and imaging assessment. Use dementia scores appropriately to identify the domains affected

↓

Step 2
Rule out pseudo-dementia and other reversible causes and treatable dementia syndromes

↓

Step 3
Assess patient eligibility for medical therapy

↓

Step 4
Periodic monitoring and follow-up

FLOWCHART 1: Approach to management of a patient with dementia.

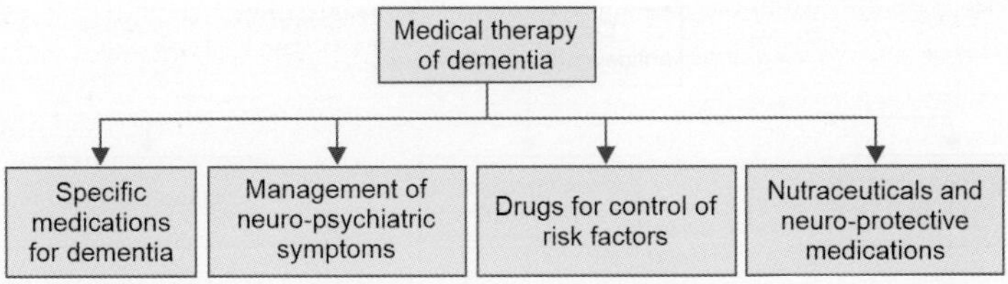

FLOWCHART 2: Medical management of a patient with dementia.

Q2. Antipsychotic for neurology practice—how to choose the right agent?

Ans. The term "organic psychosis" is used to refer to hallucinations and psychotic symptoms in the presence of an underlying pathology. Acute organic psychosis is commonly observed in individuals with metabolic derangements, febrile infection/sepsis, prolonged hospitalization/ICU stay as well as in individuals with a primary neurological illness such as stroke, neurodegenerative disorders (like Parkinson's disease and frontotemporal dementia). As neurologists we commonly encounter these patients and a basic understanding of the various antipsychotic agents is mandatory to choose the right agent and improve patient care.

Dopamine is the key neurotransmitter concerned with hallucinations and psychosis and dopaminergic dysfunction involving the meso-cortical and meso-limbic pathways is believed to play the major role (dopamine hypothesis of schizophrenia). Almost all antipsychotics work by reducing the dopaminergic activity either directly or indirectly and based on their mechanism of actions are classified as typical (1st generation) or atypical (2nd generation) antipsychotics **(Flowchart 3)**. The decision to choose the agent is based on the clinical profile of the patient and adverse drug profile of the agent. Accordingly certain medications are preferred or deferred in specific scenarios as depicted in **Table 2**.[4-7]

Q3. How to approach a patient with suspected cerebrospinal fluid (CSF) rhinorrhea?

Ans. Cerebrospinal fluid (CSF) rhinorrhea refers to abnormal leak of the CSF through the nose as result of cranial CSF leaks due to a bony defect. The major causes for CSF rhinorrhea include craniofacial trauma and cranial/endonasal surgeries. Spontaneous leak without preceding trauma or surgery can be seen in patients with increased intracranial pressure such as idiopathic intracranial hypertension (IIH), obstructive sleep apnea (OSA) and intracranial tumors. Patients typically complain of a clear watery nasal discharge. The discharge is typically clear and not sticky and has sweet/salty taste when associated with postnasal drip. Recurrent meningitis and orthostatic headache are other scenarios where CSF rhinorrhea needs to be suspected.

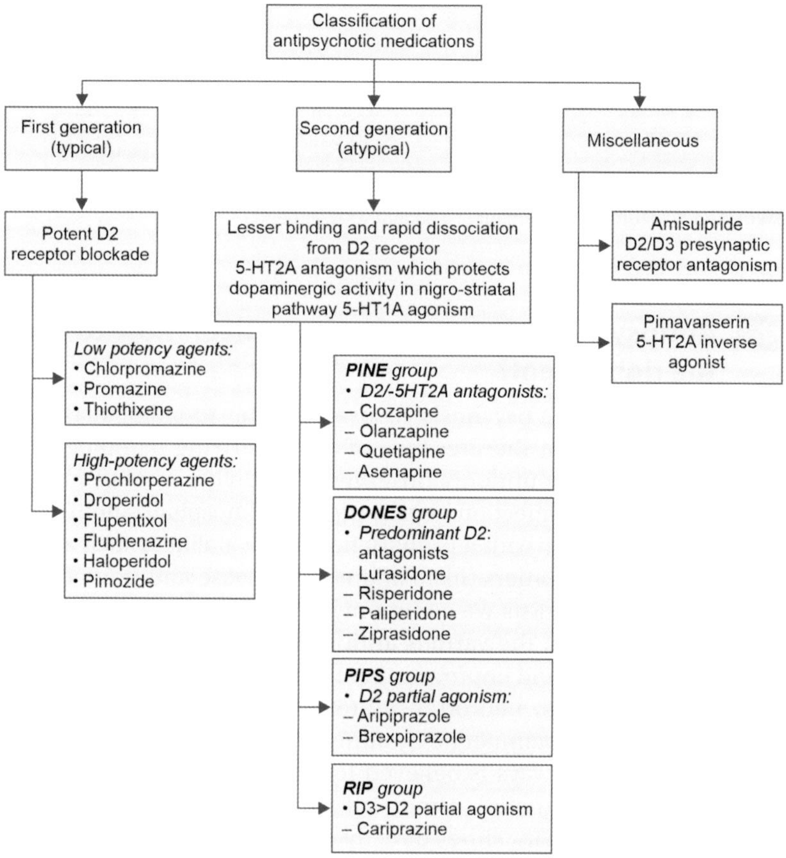

FLOWCHART 3: Classification of antipsychotic agents.

TABLE 2: Suggested choice of antipsychotic based on patient's clinical profile.

Clinical profile	Preferred agents	Agents to be avoided
Risk of acute extrapyramidal syndrome	Quetiapine, olanzapine, and aripiprazole	Typical antipsychotics
Dyslipidemia, metabolic syndrome, and hyperglycemia	Lurasidone, aripiprazole, and amisulpride	Quetiapine and olanzapine
Risk of QT prolongation	Lurasidone and aripiprazole	Quetiapine, olanzapine, and clozapine
Sedation to be minimized or avoided	Paliperidone, aripiprazole, and amisulpride	Quetiapine and olanzapine
Cytopenia and risk of bone marrow suppression		Clozapine
Coexistent hyperkinetic movement disorder	Risperidone and haloperidol	
Risk of akathisia	Quetiapine, olanzapine, and aripiprazole	Typical antipsychotics
Coexistent parkinsonism	Pimavanserin, quetiapine, olanzapine, and clozapine	Typical antipsychotics

Once suspected the first preferred investigation is to collect the fluid and assess for beta-2-transferrin by immunohistochemical assays. Beta-2-transferrin in present in CSF, perilymph, and vitreous humor. The quantity of perilymph is too less while the contamination of nasal secretions with vitreous humor is extremely rare making the presence of beta-2-transferrin in nasal discharge highly sensitive for CSF rhinorrhea (100%) with specificity ranging between 70 and 95%.

Once CSF rhinorrhea is established the next step is to look for the location of leak and plan surgical repair accordingly. Several imaging modalities are used to identify the leak and their advantages and disadvantages are summarized in **Table 3**. An algorithmic approach to suspected CSF rhinorrhea is provided in **Flowchart 4**.[8-11]

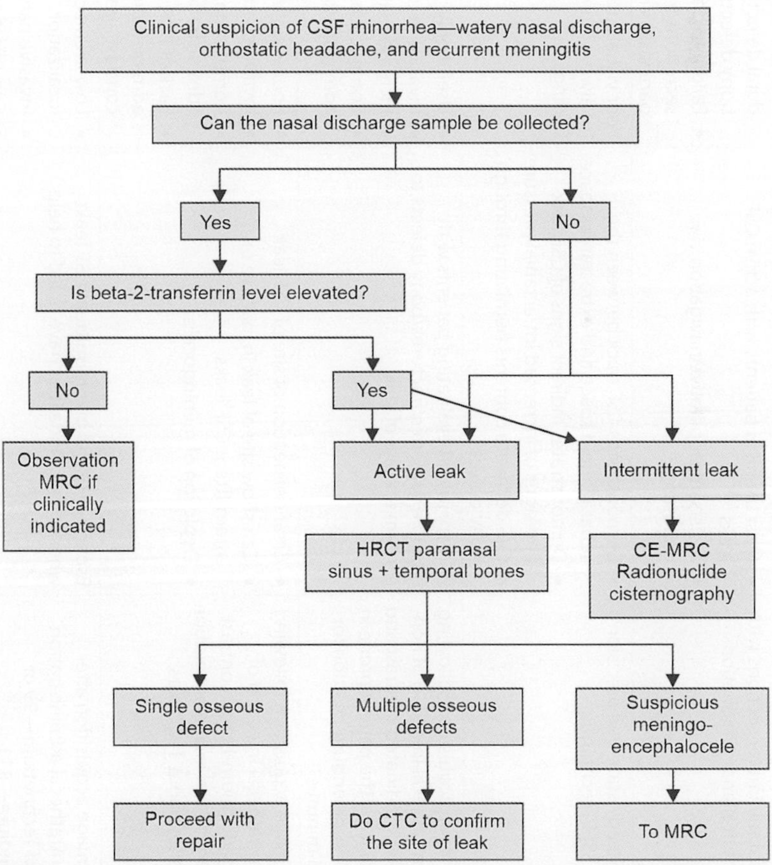

FLOWCHART 4: Algorithmic approach to a patient with suspected cerebrospinal fluid (CSF) leak.

(CE-MRC: contrast-enhanced MR cisternography; CTC: CT cisternography; MRC: MR cisternography)

TABLE 3: Various imaging modalities used in the assessment of cerebrospinal fluid (CSF) rhinorrhea.

Modality	Technique	Advantages	Disadvantages	Accuracy
Hight resolution CT (HRCT) of paranasal sinuses including temporal bones	Isotropic, volumetric, thin submillimeter sections with multiplanar reformations	• Excellent delineation of bony anatomy • Most useful in patients with active CSF leaks • Assists intraoperative navigation via endoscopy	• Failure to ascertain concomitant dural defect in the setting of multiple bony defects • Failure to differentiate mucus secretions from CSF collections in paranasal sinuses	84–95% sensitivity 57–100% specificity
MR cisternography (MRC)	Steady state free precision (SSFP) technique	• Demonstrates CSF track between the subarachnoid space and extracranial space • Demonstrates indirect signs of CSF leak and signs of increased intracranial pressure • Can delineate contents herniating through bony defect	Poor visualization of bony window (to always interpret along with HRCT findings)	94% sensitivity
CT cisternography (CTC)	Image acquisition following intrathecal injection of non-ionic iodinated contrast and placing the patient prone in Trendelenburg position for 5 minutes	Primary role in evaluating patients with multiple surgeries/fractures/bony defects to confirm the site of leak	• Useful only in active CSF leaks • Invasive nature • Increased radiation exposure • Complications related to intrathecal administration	85–92% sensitivity (in active CSF leaks) 40% sensitivity (in intermittent/ inactive CSF leaks)
Contrast-enhanced MR cisternography (CE-MRC)	Image acquisition following intrathecal injection of gadolinium-based contrast agent and image acquisition after about 1–2 hours.	• Clear delineation of site of CSF leak • Can show site of leak in inactive or intermittent CSF leaks • Depiction of meningoceles	• Poor visualization of bony window • Invasive nature • Complications related to intrathecal administration • Lack of FDA approval for intrathecal administration of the gadolinium contrast agents	92–100% sensitivity (in active CSF leaks) 70% sensitivity (in intermittent/ inactive CSF leaks) 80% specificity
Radionuclide cisternography	Image acquisition after intrathecal administration of Technetium—99 or Indium—111	Especially useful in intermittent CSF leaks where other modalities have failed to help	• Low accuracy and suboptimal localization • Invasive nature • Complications related to intrathecal administration • Complications related to exposure to radioactive agents	• Accuracy 70% in active leaks • Accuracy <28% in inactive leaks

Q4. How to evaluate for organic causes in a patient with new onset psychiatric illness?

Ans. In patients presenting with an acute or new onset neuropsychiatric dysfunction (such as psychosis/hallucinations, mood fluctuations, behavior changes, depression, and suicidal thoughts) investigations to identify underlying (organic) causes are warranted. It is not possible to do every investigation for all patients presenting with neuropsychiatric symptoms. Still a basic understanding of the psychiatric manifestations of neurological and systemic disorders helps in clinical decision-making. One major difference between the approach of a traditional neurologist and a traditional psychiatrist is that neurological illness has a one-to-one relationship between the symptomatology, pathology, and region of the nervous system which is lacking in most psychiatric illnesses.

Clinical features which suggest an underlying medical disorder in a new onset psychiatric illness include abrupt onset of symptoms, presentations in extremes of age, prominent visual hallucinations, associated neurological features such as gait dysfunction, seizures, or extrapyramidal symptoms, a clinical phenotype not fixing into a defined psychiatric syndrome, fluctuating cognition and behavior (may suggest delirium), cognitive impairment disproportionate and atypical for the psychiatric illness, fever, progressive weight loss, and high-risk behavior (substance abuse). Certain neurological disorders such as central nervous system (CNS) vasculitis and autoimmune encephalitis [anti-N-methyl-D-aspartate receptor (NMDAR) encephalitis] can have isolated psychiatric symptoms and require a high degree of clinical suspicion for further evaluation.

Some common neurological and systemic disorders and their psychiatric manifestations are summarized in **Table 4**. Over the last few years, patients with non-convulsive status epilepticus masquerading as delirium and new onset psychiatric illness have been increasingly reported. Also, the clinical spectrum of immune encephalitis (autoimmune and paraneoplastic encephalitis) is being increasingly widened to include patients with isolated psychiatric manifestations. The spectrum of neuropsychiatric manifestations reported in NMDAR encephalitis is summarized in **Box 1**.[12-16]

Q5. Discuss the management of sudomotor disorders.

Ans. Sudomotor function refers to sweat production and release which plays a key role in thermoregulation. Sweat gland is innervated by thin unmyelinated Type-C sympathetic fibers which utilize acetylcholine as the neurotransmitter. The central control for sweat production is regulated at the pre-optic anterior hypothalamus and is influenced by cortical centers and several external/internal factors. Sudomotor dysfunction is commonly encountered in small fiber neuropathies. However, diseases affecting any part of the neuraxis can lead to sudomotor dysfunction **(Flowchart 5)**.

The diagnosis of sudomotor dysfunction is complicated by the failure to demonstrate straightforward clinical findings. In most cases sudomotor

<table>
<tr><th colspan="3">TABLE 4: Neuropsychiatric manifestations of common neurological and medical disorders.</th></tr>
<tr><th colspan="2">Disorder</th><th>Psychiatric manifestations</th></tr>
<tr><td colspan="2">Traumatic brain injury</td><td>• Depression and psychosis
• Behavior changes, impulsivity, and anti-social personality
• Mood disorders, apathy
• Substance abuse
• Anhedonia, poor sleep and appetite, and chronic fatigue
• Anxiety disorder (PTSD, GAD)</td></tr>
<tr><td colspan="2">Vascular diseases of the brain
Infarct, hemorrhage</td><td>• Cognitive impairment
• Depression and dementia
• Pseudo-bulbar affect
• Anxiety disorder
• Amotivation and impaired judgement</td></tr>
<tr><td rowspan="2">Neurodegenerative disorders</td><td>PD</td><td>• Depression and anxiety
• Psychosis and hallucinations
• Impulse control disorder</td></tr>
<tr><td>Dementia syndromes</td><td>• Depression, apathy, and anxiety
• Psychosis and hallucinations
• Behavior changes, impulsivity, and anti-social personality
• Anhedonia</td></tr>
<tr><td colspan="2">Multiple sclerosis</td><td>• Demoralization and depression
• Cognitive impairment and chronic fatigue
• IEED
• Pseudobulbar affect</td></tr>
<tr><td colspan="2">Epilepsy</td><td>• Cognitive impairment
• Depression, anxiety, and mania
• Psychosis and hallucinations
• Suicidal ideation
• Forced normalization</td></tr>
<tr><td colspan="2">CNS infection/inflammation
Chronic meningitis
Viral encephalitis
CNS vasculitis
Immune mediated encephalitis
HIV/AIDS and neurosyphilis
Prion diseases
SREAT</td><td>• Delirium
• Psychosis and hallucinations
• Behavior changes, impulsivity, and anti-social personality
• Anhedonia, poor sleep and appetite, and chronic fatigue
• Cognitive impairment</td></tr>
</table>

Continued

Continued

Disorder		Psychiatric manifestations
Metabolic disorders Dyselectrolytemia Hypothyroidism Renal failure/ liver failure Acute intermittent porphyria Wilson's disease Hyperglycemia CO_2 narcosis		• Delirium • Depression and mania • Behavior changes • Psychosis and hallucinations • Apathy and anhedonia
Drugs/toxins	Medications (steroids, sympathomimetics, CNS stimulants, anti-seizure medications, and dopaminergic agonists)	• Psychosis and hallucinations • Mania • Suicidal ideation • Delirium
	Alcohol intoxication	• Psychosis • Behavior changes • Delirium tremens • Addiction and withdrawal features
	Recreational agents (cannabis, cocaine, marijuana, LSD, and hallucinogens)	• Psychosis and hallucinations • Mania • Suicidal ideation • Delirium • Depression • Anti-social behavior
	Heavy metal toxicity (lead, mercury, and arsenic)	• Psychosis and hallucinations • Mania • Delirium

(AIDS: acquired immunodeficiency syndrome; CNS: central nervous system; GAD: generalized anxiety disorder; HIV: human immunodeficiency virus; IEED: involuntary emotional expression disorder; LSD: lysergic acid diethylamide; PD: Parkinson's disease; PTSD: post-traumatic stress disorder; SREAT: steroid-responsive encephalopathy associated with autoimmune thyroiditis)

BOX 1: Diagnostic clues and spectrum of clinical presentation of anti-N-methyl-D-aspartate receptor (NMDAR) encephalitis.

- *S*leep dysfunction
- *E*xcitement, disinhibition, or manic behavior alternating with depressive behavior
- *A*ggression and/or agitation
- *R*apid onset
- *C*hildren and young adult predominant involvement
- *H*istory of no prior psychiatric disease
- *F*luctuating catatonia
- *N*egative and positive symptoms at presentation
- *M*emory impairment
- *D*ecrease in verbal output/mutism
- *A*ntipsychotic intolerance
- *R*igidity, hyperthermia, and coma similar to neuroleptic malignant syndrome
- Antibody in serum or CSF

Mnemonic—SEARCH for NMDAR antibody

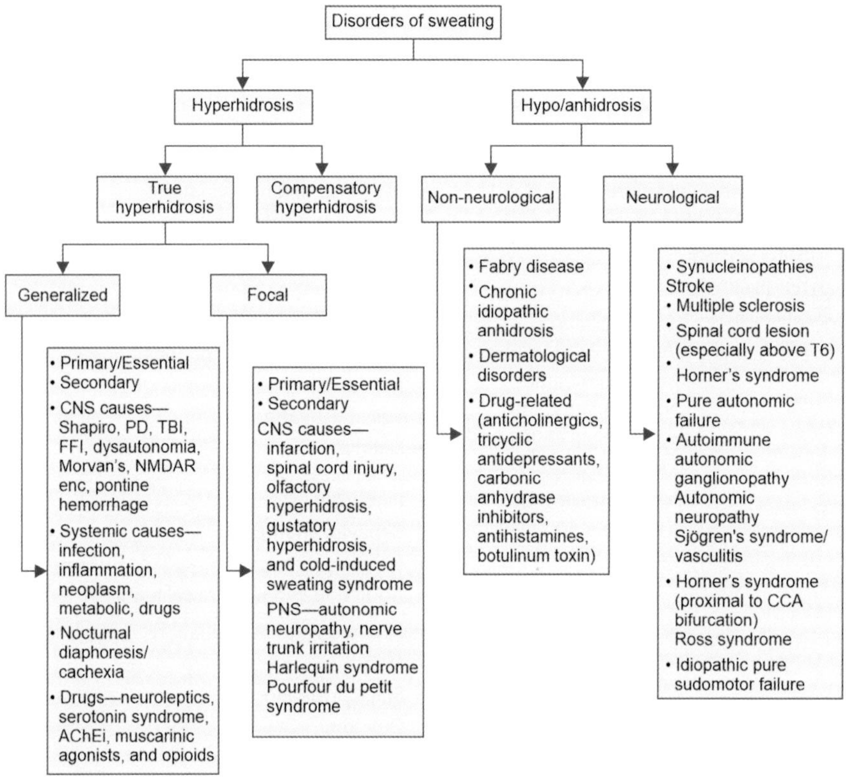

FLOWCHART 5: Classification of sudomotor disorders.

(AChEi: acetylcholinesterase inhibitors; CCA: common carotid artery; FFI: fatal familial insomnia; PD: Parkinson's disease; TBI: traumatic brain injury)

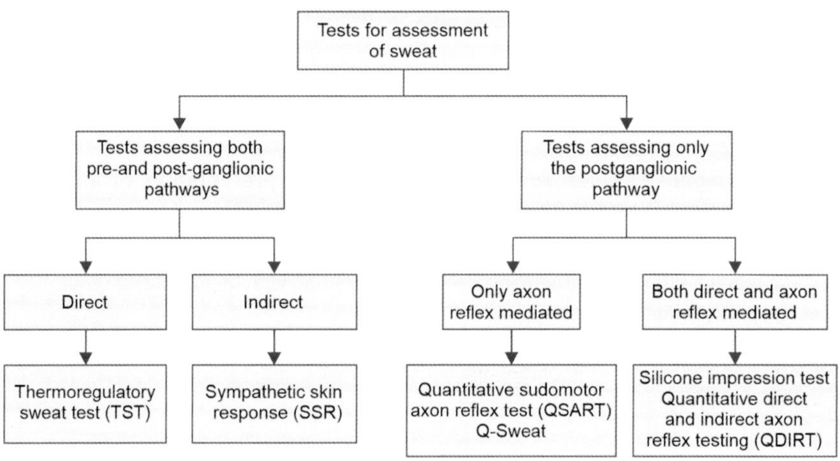

FLOWCHART 6: Tests for assessment of sweating.

dysfunction is a part of the neurological illness. Specialized demonstration of sudomotor function (or dysfunction) can be achieved by the use of specialized diagnostic modalities **(Flowchart 6 and Table 5)**.

TABLE 5: Summary of the various diagnostic modalities for assessment of sweating.

	TST	SSR	QSART	Silicone impression	QDIRT
Stimulus	Whole body heating	Electrical current delivered to a peripheral sensory nerve	Iontophoresis of acetylcholine	Iontophoresis of pilocarpine or acetylcholine	Iontophoresis of acetylcholine
Response	Anatomic distribution of sweating over the anterior body surface	Change in electrodermal potential over the palms or soles	Latency, magnitude, and duration of sudomotor output in the four limb sites	Size and number of individual sweat droplets over a defined area of skin	• Similar to QSART • No requirement of sweat capsule • Sweat production photographed after application of dye–alizarin red
Site of lesion detection	Pre and post ganglionic	Pre and post ganglionic	Post ganglionic axonal only	Post ganglionic direct and axonal	Post ganglionic direct and axonal
Sudomotor assessment	Direct	Indirect	Direct	Direct	Direct
Need for specialized equipment	Yes	No	Yes	Yes	Yes
Objectivity	Poor	Good	Good	Good	Good
Standardized procedure	Yes	Yes	Yes	No	No
Time consumption	60–120 minutes	5 minutes	15–20 minutes	15 minutes	15 minutes
Technical interference	Low (manual calculation)	Very high	Low (correct marking)	High (proper placement)	Very low
Repeatability/ reproducibility	Yes	Poor (habituate)	Yes	Yes	Yes
Sampling sites	Excellent	Limited	Limited	Limited –may be better	Limited –may be better

(QDIRT: quantitative direct and indirect axon reflex testing; QSART: quantitative sudomotor axon reflex test; SSR: sympathetic skin response; TST: thermoregulatory sweat test)

TABLE 6: Treatment modalities for sudomotor dysfunction (hyperhidrosis).	
Local modalities	• Antiperspirants (aluminum chloride 15–25%) • Tap water iontophoresis (for palmar/plantar sweating) • Botulinum toxin injection
Systemic medications	• Anticholinergic drugs (glycopyrrolate) • Tricyclic antidepressants (amitriptyline) • Beta blockers • Centrally acting sympatholytic drugs (clonidine) • Calcium channel blockers (diltiazem)
Surgical interventions	• Endoscopic thoracic sympathectomy in sweating–disorders of the upper quadrant • Axillary curettage, liposuction for axillary hyperhidrosis

Management of sudomotor dysfunction involves identification of the underlying disorder and directed therapies specific to the underlying etiology. In addition, complications related to sudomotor dysfunction and trophic changes need special care and attention. The various treatment modalities for hyperhidrosis are summarized in **Table 6**. The management options for hypo/anhidrosis are limited. Patients may be encouraged to use moisturizer, avoid agents such as anticholinergics/antihistaminergics which can further worsen the hypo/anhidrosis, and perform exertional activities in a cool, well-ventilated environment. In patients with autoimmune neuropathy and acquired idiopathic generalized anhidrosis (AIGA) steroid therapy may be beneficial.[17-23]

Q6. Discuss the role of vestibular sedatives for common vestibular disorders—BPPV, vestibular migraine, and PPPD.

Ans. Vertigo is a commonly observed neurological symptom where the patient perceives a feeling of movement, a sensation as if the external world were revolving around the patient (objective vertigo) or as if he himself were revolving in space (subjective vertigo). Several diseases can lead to vertigo and these are broadly classified into central and peripheral causes **(Table 7)**.

The commonly used medication for acute vertigo/vestibular syndrome includes the vestibular sedative agents and antiemetic agents **(Table 8)**. These agents are most useful in acute setting and provide early symptomatic relief without altering the underlying pathophysiology. In fact, prolonged use of vestibular sedatives is not recommended as it tends to affect the central adaptive mechanisms. Robust data exists regarding the use of vestibular sedatives in patients with vestibular neuritis and acute vestibular hypofunctioning. The role of vestibular sedatives in select disorders such as benign paroxysmal positional vertigo (BPPV), vestibular migraine, and persistent postural-perceptual dizziness (PPPD) is unknown.

TABLE 7: Central and peripheral causes of vertigo.

Central causes	Peripheral causes
• Posterior circulation strokes • Posterior fossa tumors • Brainstem/cerebellar demyelination • Epilepsy • Vestibular migraine • Rhombencephalitis • Persistent postural-perceptual dizziness (PPPD)	• Benign paroxysmal positional vertigo (BPPV) • Vestibular neuritis • Labyrinthitis • Ménière's disease • Superior semicircular canal (SCC) dehiscence • Otosclerosis

TABLE 8: Common medications used in the management of vertigo.

Drug class	Common agents	Dosing schedule	Adverse effects
Antihistamines	Meclizine	25–50 mg thrice daily (oral)	• Sedation • Fatigue • Blurred vision
	Promethazine	15–25 mg oral, IM or rectal administration	• Sedation • EPS
	Dimenhydrinate	50–100 mg thrice daily (oral)	• Sedation • Blurred vision
Anticholinergics	Scopolamine	• 0.6 mg four times a day • Also available as transdermal patch	• Sedation • Dry mouth • Urinary retention • Can worsen acute angle closure glaucoma
Histamine agonists	Betahistine	48–96 mg daily in divided doses	• Gastritis • Only non-sedating vestibular suppressant
Calcium channel blocker	Cinnarizine	25–75 mg, twice or thrice daily (oral)	• Sedation pedal edema and weight gain • EPS
Benzodiazepines	Diazepam	2–5 mg oral or IV once or twice daily	• Sedation, addiction • Slurred speech
	Lorazepam	0.5–2 mg oral, IM or IV administration once every 4–8 hours	
	Clonazepam	0.25–1 mg, once or twice daily	

Continued

Continued

Drug class	Common agents	Dosing schedule	Adverse effects
Antiemetic agents	Metoclopramide	5–10 mg oral or IV every 4–6 hours	• Sedation • EPS/acute dystonic reaction • Atrioventricular block • Bradycardia • Bronchospasm, Drowsiness • Gynecomastia • Tardive dyskinesia
	Prochlorperazine	5–10 mg oral or IM every 4–6 hours	• Agitation • Dizziness • Photosensitivity • EPS
	Ondansetron	4 mg IV or oral thrice/day	• Headache • Diarrhea
(EPS: extrapyramidal syndrome; IM: intramuscular; IV: intravenous)			

TABLE 9: Diagnostic provocative maneuvers and canal repositioning maneuvers for various benign paroxysmal positional vertigo (BPPV) syndromes.

BPPV syndrome	Diagnostic provocative maneuvers	Canal repositioning maneuvers
Posterior canal (PC) BPPV	Dix-Hallpike test	• Modified Epley maneuver • Semont liberatory maneuver
Horizontal canal (HC) BPPV	• Supine roll test • Bow and lean test	• Barbeque roll maneuver • Gufoni maneuver
Anterior/superior canal (HC) BPPV	Dix-Hallpike test (reverse of PC BPPV)	• Reverse Epley/reverse Semont maneuver • Deep head hanging maneuver

The primary treatment of BPPV is canal repositioning maneuver (CRM) based on the side and semicircular canal affected. The diagnosis of BPPV is clinical. The various provocative maneuvers and CRM for the different BPPV are summarized in **Table 9**. A recent meta-analysis by Sharif S et al. published in 2023, which included six randomized controlled trials (RCT) concluded that there is no role for vestibular sedatives in BPPV and the use of vestibular sedatives may be associated with increased adverse effects and reduced sensitivity of diagnostic maneuvers which tend to affect the canal repositioning maneuvers leading to inadequate symptom control. The expert opinion, however, suggests a possible short-term role of vestibular sedatives for 2–3 days in select patients with residual symptoms in spite of CRM or those too anxious to undergo CRM.

Vestibular migraine is a complex neurological disorder and the diagnosis is essentially clinical. Some patients have isolated vertigo/vestibular symptoms with no concomitant headache making diagnosis challenging. A reasonable exclusion of alternative etiologies including BPPV and other peripheral causes is warranted. Currently there is no evidence to recommend the role of vestibular sedatives in patients with vestibular migraine. In the acute phase, antiemetics can be used to help relieve the vertigo and vestibular symptoms. Studies have shown that migraine abortive medications such as triptans improve the vertiginous symptoms. In the chronic phases migraine preventive medications (propranolol, valproic acid, flunarizine, amitriptyline etc.) in addition to vestibular rehabilitation therapy (VRT) help improving activities of daily living and reduce symptom recurrence. Long term or continuous use of vestibular sedatives is not recommended.

Persistent postural-perceptual dizziness is a relatively recent disorder described since 2017. It is classified as a chronic vestibular disorder and is closely associated with migraine and neuropsychiatric conditions such as depression and anxiety. The diagnosis of PPPD is essentially clinical with reasonable exclusion of alternative pathologies. The mainstay of treatment in PPPD is cognitive behavior therapy (CBT), addressing psychiatric comorbidities, and VRT. Several studies have demonstrated the benefit of antidepressive medications (SSRIs and SNRIs) in improving the symptoms of PPPD. Currently no data or recommendations exist favoring the use of vestibular sedatives in PPPD and similar to other chronic vestibular disorders long term use of vestibular sedatives is not recommended.[24-30]

Q7. Discuss the approach to visual hallucinations in adults.

Ans. Visual hallucination is visualizing something which is not present, that is a visual percept without a stimulus.[31] Visual hallucination can be simple—perceiving geometrical patterns or complex—perceiving animals or people.[31] Visual hallucinations can be ophthalmological as in people with visual loss or neurological as in diseases such as Parkinson's disease and dementia with Lewy body disease **(Flowchart 7)**. Drugs and psychiatric illnesses can present with visual hallucination. The different conditions associated with visual hallucination, the neural networks involved, the neurotransmitters associated with it and the treatment approach is discussed here.[32,33]

Pathogenesis of Visual Hallucinations

- Absence of visual input
- Impaired visual information processing
- Over activation of default mode network[32]
- Impaired activity of dorsal attention network
- Thalamus, a diencephalic hub of sensory processing is also a driver of neural networks
- The thalamocortical dysrhythmia resulting in improper shifting of brain networks

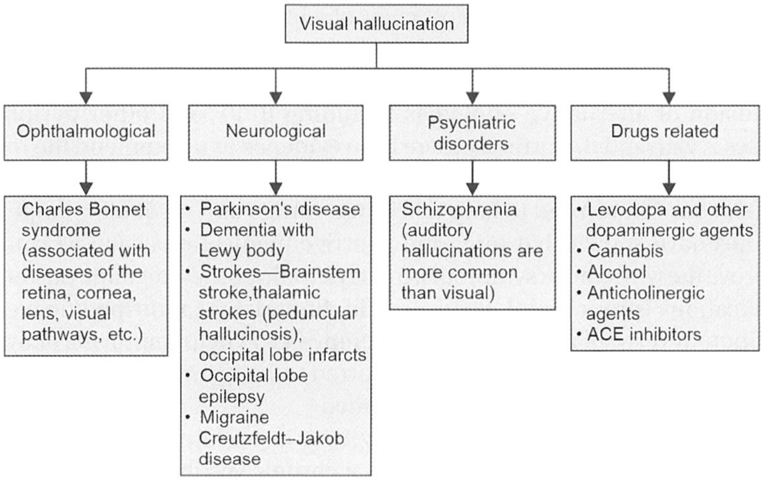

FLOWCHART 7: Classification of subtypes of visual hallucination.

- Hodo-topic approach toward neural substrates and networks are needed to conceptualize the exact mechanism[34]
- The three models—perception attentional dysfunction model, deafferentation hyperexcitability model, misattribution of internal imagery model—are implicated.[32]

Neurotransmitters

- Reduced cholinergic function
- Reduction in GABA activity
- Involvement of 5-hydroxytryptamine 2A binding[32]
- Dopamine has a complex role in the genesis of visual hallucinations in Parkinsonism
- Levodopa therapy potentially enhances the genesis of visual hallucinations

Treatment (Table 10)

- Lighting the home well in the evening
- Cholinesterase inhibitors[34]
    - Rivastigmine
    - Galantamine
    - Donepezil
    - Memantine
- 5-HT 2A antagonist/inverse agonist
    - Clozapine
    - Pimavanserin
    - Quetiapine
    - Olanzapine
- Repetitive transcranial magnetic stimulation (rTMS)[34]
- Transcranial direct electrical stimulation (TCdES)

TABLE 10: Treatment of various types of visual hallucinations.

Disease	Type	Clinical features	Treatment	Specific remarks
Charles Bonnet syndrome	Ophthalmological due to visual impairment	Simple hallucination, colors, and geometrical patterns	Self-help techniques—eye movements, increasing brightness 5-HT antagonists	SSRI Yi-Gan San (a traditional Chinese drug with multi neurotransmitter effect) rTMS
Parkinson's disease	Neurological	Presence hallucinations and passage hallucinations	Reduction in PD medication Clozapine Olanzapine Quetiapine	While reducing the PD medication, dopamine withdrawal syndrome and neuroleptic malignant syndrome to be kept in mind
Dementia with Lewy bodies[31]	Neurological	Minor and complex	Donepezil Memantine Galantamine Rivastigmine	Complex visual hallucinations are associated with cognitive impairment. Anti-psychotics to be used with caution.
Migraine	Neurological	Zig zag lines, flash of lights, fortification spectra, and scintillating scotomas	Anti-migraine prophylaxis	Associated nausea, vomiting, and photo/phonophobia
Occipital epilepsy	Neurological	Elementary visual hallucinations	Anti-seizure medication	Confined to hemifield, stereotypical lasting for a few seconds. May increase in size mostly circular
Creutzfeldt-Jakob disease	Neurological	Cognitive decline and myoclonic jerks.		Cortical ribbon sign and pulvinar sign in MRI

Continued

Continued

Disease	Type	Clinical features	Treatment	Specific remarks
Strokes	Neurological	Brainstem and thalamic strokes Peduncular hallucinosis	Treatment as per stroke protocol	Visuo-acoustic and visuo-tactile
Sleep related[33]	Neurological	Hypnogogic and hypnopompic hallucinations	Treatment of underlying narcolepsy.	These occur in the borders of sleep mostly in narcolepsy.
Schizophrenia	Psychiatry	Auditory hallucinations are more common than visual	Typical and atypical anti-psychotics	–
Levodopa	Drugs	Visual hallucinations are primarily nocturnal, non-threatening, and unique in each patient	Down titration of levodopa, quetiapine, and olanzapine	Very bothersome for the caregivers
Cannabis	Drugs	Associated altered perception, spiritual and mystical content	Stop the offending drug	Nine tetrahydrocannabinol (THC) is the active constituent.
Ethanol toxicity/ withdrawal	Drugs	Multimodal hallucinations	Ethanol withdrawal treatment as per protocol	Delirium tremens-white mice hallucinations Unpleasant mostly
Drugs	ACE inhibitors Anticholinergics Amantadine Baclofen withdrawal	Multimodal hallucinations with psycho active content depending upon the hallucinogen	Stop or down titrate the offending drug In case of baclofen pump failure replace baclofen	To be cautious in intrathecal baclofen pump failure

Q8. Discuss the approach to a patient with problems of sleep initiation.

Ans. Diagnostic and Statistical Manual of Mental Disorders, Fifth Edition (DSM-V) defines insomnia as a sleep disorder characterized by difficulty in sleep initiation and/or sleep maintenance, occurring at least 3 times per week for at least 3 months, causing significant personal distress, and associated with daytime functional impairments. Insomnia is seen in 10–40% adult population according to most studies. The major causes of insomnia are summarized in **Box 2**. Unaddressed insomnia can lead to mood disorder, emotional distress, irritability, impaired concentration, fatigue, and disturbances in social and interpersonal relationships. Insomnia is broadly divided into acute/short-term insomnia (symptoms <3 months) and chronic (symptoms >3 months).

Insomnia is a clinical diagnosis and assessment of sleep history is essential. Patients should be instructed to maintain a sleep diary **(Box 3)** to help

BOX 2: Common causes of insomnia.

- *I*llness secondary to underlying medical condition
- *N*eurological disorders and psychiatric illness
- *S*leep disorders (primary)
- *O*verconcern about lack of sleep
- *M*edication-related sleep impairment
- *N*oisy and/or unpleasant/uncomfortable sleep environment
- *I*diopathic
- *A*nxiety disorder
- *C*ircadian rhythm disturbance/disruption

Mnemonic—*INSOMNIAC*

BOX 3: Components of sleep diary.

- Time to go to bed
- Time falling asleep
- Time taken to fall asleep
- Number of sleep interruptions/awakenings
- Duration of sleep interruptions/awakenings
- Time of final awakening
- Time spent in bed after final awakening
- Was the final awakening earlier or later than the intended time of awakening
- Total sleep duration
- Rating the quality of sleep subjectively
- The feeling of refreshed sleep
- Number of daytime naps/dozes
- Consumptions of caffeine or alcohol
- Consumption of drugs or substances for sleep

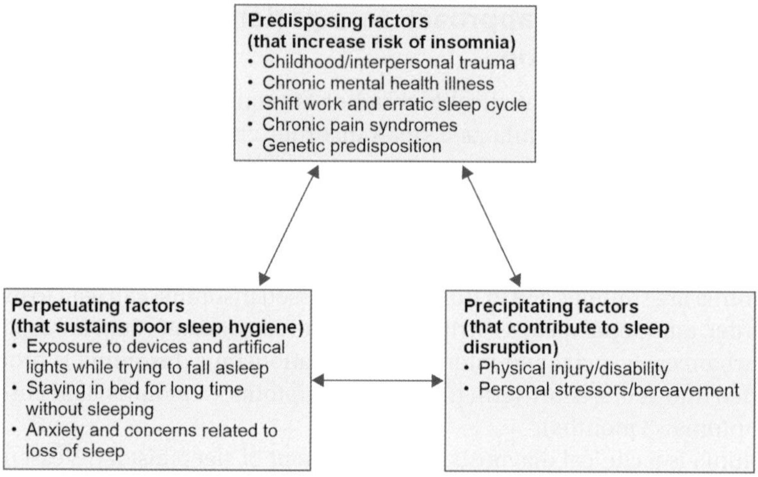

FIG. 1: 3P model for insomnia.

identify factors contributing to poor sleep hygiene. Validated questionnaires such as the *Pittsburgh Sleep Quality Index* and Sleep Problems Questionnaire help characterize symptom severity and assist in monitoring response during follow-up. Current guidelines do not recommend polysomnography routinely in all patients with chronic insomnia unless a coexistent sleep disorder (such as obstructive sleep apnea or periodic limb movement disorder) is suspected. Actigraphy is an inexpensive tool that acts as a surrogate marker of sleep and wakefulness and can be used along with a sleep diary.

Insomnia is now viewed as an independent sleep disorder with two core conceptual frameworks to help understand the disease process and guide cognitive behavior therapy (CBT). The 3P model conceptualizes the various comorbid behavior and conditions that contribute to insomnia **(Fig. 1)**. Conditioned arousal and sleep-related hyperarousal model propose that a conditioned response to sleep environment contributes to insomnia.

Management of a patient with insomnia requires a combination of pharmacological and non-pharmacological modalities tailored as per the clinical profile **(Table 11)**, in addition to avoidance/addressing underlying medical and psychiatric comorbid illness. Benzodiazepines with their longer half-lives have a higher risk of dependence and habituation and are associated with adverse safety profile. Because of these reasons non-benzodiazepine agents are preferred in the management of chronic insomnia.[35-39]

Q9. Discuss the approach to a patient with daytime somnolence.

Ans. Excessive daytime sleepiness/somnolence (EDS) is a commonly encountered symptom and studies have demonstrated that up to 33% of adults experience EDS at some point in time leading to significant functional impairment. The common comorbid conditions associated with EDS include

TABLE 11: Management of insomnia.

Non-pharmacological management of insomnia	CBT	*Components of CBT*
		• Sleep education • Sleep restriction therapy • Sleep compression • Stimulus control therapy • Cognitive therapy • Sleep hygiene • Counter-arousal measures (PMR and diaphragmatic breathing)
Pharmacological management of insomnia	Non-benzodiazepine BZRAs	• Zolpidem • Zaleplon • Zopiclone • Eszopiclone
	DORA	• Lemborexant • Suvorexant • Daridorexant
	Melatonin/agonists	• Melatonin • Ramelteon
	Tricyclic antidepressants	• Doxepin • Amitriptyline
	Other antidepressants	• Trazodone • Mirtazapine
	Antipsychotics	• Quetiapine
	Hypnotic Benzodiazepines	• Estazolam • Flurazepam • Quazepam • Temazepam (safest) • Triazolam
	Anxiolytic Benzodiazepines	• Clonazepam • Lorazepam • Alprazolam *Use not recommended for chronic insomnia*

(BZRA: benzodiazepine receptor agonists; CBT: cognitive behavior therapy; DORA: dual orexin receptor antagonist)

obstructive sleep apnea (OSA), primary sleep disorders, and psychiatric illness. Patients with EDS complain of episodes of falling asleep inadvertently, sleep attacks, sleep inertia, need for recurrent naps during the day, and unrefreshing night sleep. The common disorders associated with EDS are summarized in **Flowchart 8**.

An important caveat in the assessment of a patient with EDS is to differentiate sleepiness from fatigue and significant subjective overlap exists

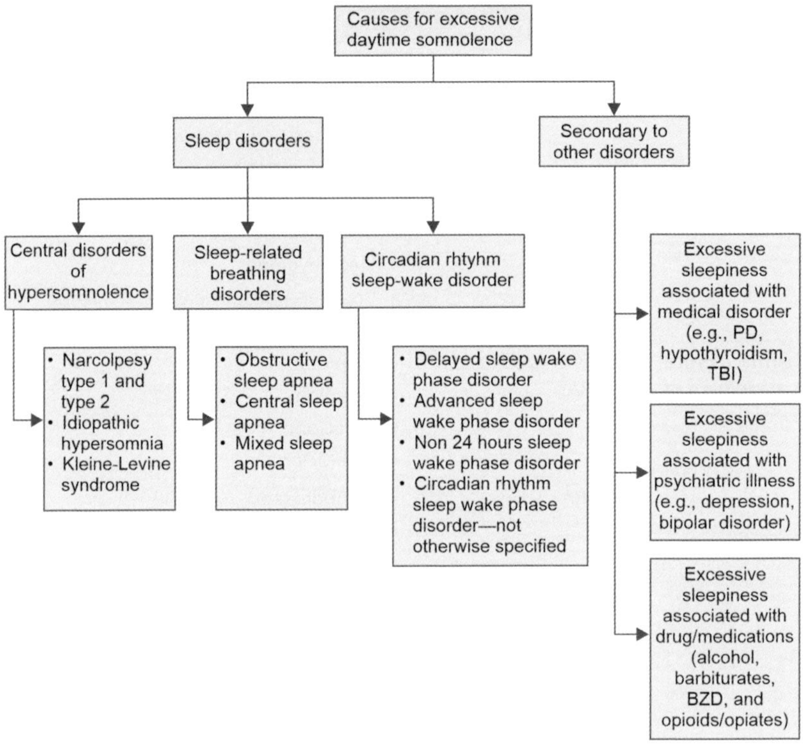

FLOWCHART 8: Disorders associated with excessive daytime somnolence (EDS).

between these two symptoms. A thorough history of the sleep pattern, history of consumption of medications (or recreational agents), and presence of other underlying medical illnesses need to be elicited in addition to enquiring bed-partner for witnessed apnea or parasomnias. The Epworth Sleepiness Scale is a validated tool to assess for EDS with a score ≥12 suggesting excessive sleepiness. Clinical examination specifically to look for oral/craniofacial abnormalities that may contribute to sleep apnea needs to be assessed. STOP-BANG questionnaire is a simple tool used for OSA screening. The approach to a patient with EDS is summarized in **Flowchart 9**. Specific diagnostic modalities available for the assessment of sleep disorders and hypersomnia are summarized in **Table 12**.

Management of EDS involves the identification and correction of underlying causes. In patients with OSA, proper utilization of continuous positive airway pressure (CPAP) improves night sleep and reduces EDS. Lifestyle changes, optimization of sedative medications, sleep hygiene, cognitive behavior therapy to improve sleep quality, and optimal management of concomitant medical disorders that can lead to EDS are the primary treatment modalities. In patients who continue to experience EDS in spite of these aforementioned steps, medications can be administered **(Table 13)**.[40-46]

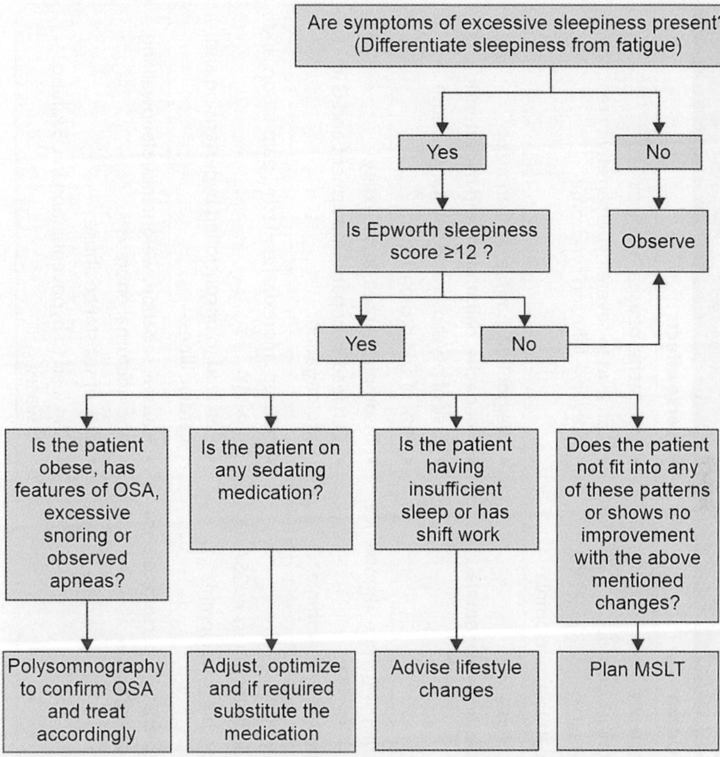

FLOWCHART 9: Approach to a patient with excessive daytime somnolence (EDS).

(MSLT: mean sleep latency test; OSA: obstructive sleep apnea) (MSLT: mean sleep latency test; OSA: obstructive sleep apnea)

TABLE 12: Diagnostic modalities for assessment of sleep disorders and hypersomnia.

Diagnostic modality	Description	Application
Actigraphy	Inexpensive surrogate wristwatch-like devices that measure movements as surrogate markers of sleep and wakefulness	• Basic screening modality for sleep assessment. • An average daily sleep time >660 minutes is suggestive of idiopathic hypersomnia. • Tends to over or underestimate the wake and sleep time.
Polysomnography (PSG)	Multimodal sleep and breathing abnormality monitoring using sensors that provide information on EEG, EOG, ECG, limb and chest movements, pulse oximetry, snoring, and body position	• Gold standard for identifying sleep-related breathing disorders • Useful to identify periodic limb movements of sleep, rapid eye movement (REM) sleep behavior disorder and parasomnias.
Mean sleep latency test (MSLT)	Patient is provided 4–5 nap opportunities at 2-hour intervals to measure the propensity and time taken to fall asleep	• Gold standard for assessment of excessive daytime somnolence. • A median sleep latency of <5 minutes is objective indication of excessive sleepiness (normal value >8–10 minutes) • Confirms narcolepsy by the presence of two or more sleep onset REM (SOREMs).

TABLE 13: Medications used in the management of hypersomnolence disorders.

Drug	Mechanism	Dosage	Indication	Adverse effects
Modafinil	Unknown	200–400 mg in the morning/before shift	Narcolepsy Shift work disorder Residual sleepiness in OSA Idiopathic hypersomnia	• Headache, nausea, anorexia • Can lead to severe hypersensitivity reaction/ Stevens–Johnson syndrome
Armodafinil	Unknown	120–250 mg in the morning/before shift		
Methylphenidate Amphetamine	Sympathomimetic agents	100 mg/day (maximum recommended dose)	Narcolepsy Idiopathic hypersomnia	• Weight loss, nausea, and anorexia • Headache, palpitation, and hypertension • Risk of psychosis and substance abuse • Risk of QTc prolongation.
Pitolisant	He receptor inverse agonist	8.9 mg/day starting dose Can go up to 17.8–35.9 mg/day	Narcolepsy (hyper-somnolence and cataplexy) Idiopathic hypersomnia	• Insomnia, nausea, and anxiety • Can lead to hepatic impairment and QTc prolongation.
Solriamfetol	Dopamine/ norepinephrine reuptake inhibitor	Start at 37.5–75 mg/day Maximum dose 150 mg/ day	Narcolepsy Residual sleepiness in OSA Idiopathic hypersomnia	• Nausea, anorexia, headache, palpitation, and anxiety. • Can lead to uncontrolled hypertension and cardiac illness
Sodium oxybate	GABA-B receptor antagonism	6–9 g/day (in divided doses)	Narcolepsy (hypersomnolence and cataplexy)	• Nausea, sedation, weight loss, sleepwalking, and nocturnal enuresis • Risk of substance abuse. • Can lead to hypoventilation in OSA/lung disease.

Q10. Discuss the approach and management of ischemic stroke with hemorrhagic transformation.

Ans. Hemorrhagic transformation (HT) refers to a spectrum of ischemia-related brain hemorrhage which is most commonly seen following intravenous thrombolysis. HT is also observed spontaneously in massive cerebral infarcts. HT is believed to be seen in 3–40% of cases of cerebral infarction and most of them go unnoticed.

A variety of classifications have been proposed to define HT. The two common classifications used are the clinical and radiological classification of HT.

Clinically HTs are classified as symptomatic or asymptomatic. Symptomatic HT is defined as a worsening of the National Institutes of Health Stroke Scale (NIHSS) by ≥4 points within the first 36 hours of stroke onset that is attributable to the hemorrhage.

Radiologically HT is defined as per the ECASS trial protocol which defined a spectrum of HT. The Heidelberg Classification Scale **(Table 14)** further extrapolates the bleeding spectrum to include every type of intracranial hemorrhage following cerebral infarction and or following reperfusion therapy.

Hemorrhagic transformation following a cerebral infarction is not necessarily bad. In fact, it is reported that mild-to-moderate HTs represent successful treatment and vessel revascularization. The principles in the management of HT are summarized in **Table 15**. HI 1, HI 2, and PH 1 are almost always associated with no major changes in morbidity or mortality. PH 2 on the other hand can be associated with a significant neurological deterioration and higher mortality.[47-51]

TABLE 14: Heidelberg classification of intracranial hemorrhage following cerebral infarction.

Class	Type	Description		Antiplatelet therapy
1. *Hemorrhagic transformation of infarcted brain tissue*	1a (HI 1)	Scattered small petechiae with no mass effect	Represents hemorrhagic transformation	Antiplatelets may be continued
	1b (HI 2)	Confluent petechiae with no mass effect		
2. *Intracerebral hemorrhage within and beyond infarcted brain tissue*	1c (PH 1)	Hematoma within infarcted tissue occupying <30% of the volume with no significant mass effect	Represents hemorrhagic transformation	Antiplatelets may be continued
	PH 2	Hematoma occupying ≥30% of infarcted brain tissue with obvious mass effect		*Antiplatelets to be withheld*
3. *Intracranial hemorrhage remote from the cerebral infarction*	3a	Remote parenchymal hematoma	Does not represent hemorrhagic transformation	
	3b	Intraventricular hemorrhage		
	3c	Subarachnoid hemorrhage		
	3d	Subdural hemorrhage		

TABLE 15: Management of hemorrhagic transformation.

Management of hemorrhagic transformation	

Preventive therapy	• Ensuring optimal selection of patients with acute cerebral infarction for revascularization therapy.
	• Usage of right dose of intravenous thrombolytic agent
	• Ensuring optimal control of hyperglycemia with a target CBG levels being <180 mg/dL (SHINE trial and GIST UK trial)
	• Optimal BP management
	  ○ Maintain systolic blood pressure (SBP) and diastolic blood pressure (DBP) <220 mm Hg and <140 mm Hg respectively in patients not eligible for thrombolysis
	  ○ Maintain SBP and DBP <180 mm Hg and <105 mm Hg respectively in patients eligible for intravenous thrombolysis
	  ○ The exact BP target for patients who undergo mechanical thrombectomy for acute stroke is yet to be established, however this value is much lower than the thrombolysis group
	• Cardio-embolic strokes are at a significantly higher risk of undergoing HT and the timing of the initiation of anticoagulant therapy is crucial to prevent HT
	  ○ AHA/ASA recommends initiation of anticoagulants 4–14 days after the acute event.
	  ○ ESC/EHRA recommends the "1-3-6-12" rule based on the NIHSS of the incident stroke (Diener's rule).
	  ○ Where possible, novel oral anticoagulants (NOACs) are preferred as they have a lower risk of HT compared to vitamin K antagonists (VKA)

Management of bleed following thrombolysis	• Achieve target BP control
	• Stop infusion of thrombolytic agents
	• Reversal of coagulopathy
	  ○ Cryoprecipitate (10 U standard dose, additional doses to be given to achieve serum fibrinogen levels >150 mg/dL)
	  ○ Platelet infusion (most useful in patients with platelet counts <100000/micL. *Routine use in other symptomatic HT controversial*)
	  ○ Prothrombin complex concentrate— Prothrombin complex concentrate (PCC) (Useful in warfarin-related IC bleed. Used as an adjunct in symptomatic HT who have received cryoprecipitate. *Isolated usage of PCC without increasing fibrinogen levels is not justified*)
	  ○ Fresh frozen plasma—FFP (*role controversial*). Maybe used as an adjunct or as a replacement of cryoprecipitate, when not available. 12 mL/kg is the British Committee for Standards in Hematology recommendation for thrombolysis-related IC bleed)
	  ○ Vitamin K (*role controversial*). May have a role in patients who are already on oral vitamin K antagonists)

Continued

Continued

<table>
<tr><th colspan="2">Management of hemorrhagic transformation</th></tr>
<tr><td></td><td>○ Antifibrinolytic agents—epsilon aminocaproic acid and tranexamic acid (no significant data). Maybe considered in all patients with symptomatic HT in adjunct to other blood products or in people who refuse blood products. Guidelines from British Committee for Standards in Hematology suggest the use of antifibrinolytic agents for treating IC bleed (in the setting of thrombolytic therapy)
○ Activated factor VII (no major data). Most studies have demonstrated an increased risk of thrombotic events following administration of this agent)
• Neurosurgical intervention—decompressive hemicraniectomy and hematoma evacuation.</td></tr>
<tr><td>Management of HT in patients receiving antiplatelets</td><td>• Antiplatelet cessation
○ In patients with symptomatic HT irrespective of imaging finding antiplatelet cessation is warranted
○ In patients whose CT shows HI 1, HI 2, or PH 1 antiplatelet therapy may be continued
○ In patients with PH 2 antiplatelet cessation is warranted
• Role of platelet transfusion is unclear
• Control of hypertension and hyperglycemia
• Neurosurgical intervention—decompressive hemicraniectomy and hematoma evacuation.</td></tr>
<tr><td>Management of HT in patients receiving anticoagulants</td><td>• Most authors follow the same principle as applied to antiplatelet agents (HI 1, HI 2, and PH 1 require no drugs cessation)
• In patients with HT of PH 2 type or symptomatic HT, anticoagulants need to be stopped and need for reversal to be decided on an individual basis
○ Vitamin K antagonists are reversed with PCC and/or vitamin K administration
○ Direct oral anticoagulants are reversed using either specific or non-specific agents
- Specific agents: Idarucizumab (monoclonal antibody against dabigatran), Andexanet alpha (modified protein similar to factor X), ciraparantag (synthetic molecule competitively binding to NOAC)
- Non-specific agents: PCC, fresh frozen plasma (FFP) and recombinant factor VIIa
• Neurosurgical intervention—decompressive hemicraniectomy and hematoma evacuation.</td></tr>
<tr><td>Experimental agents and drugs in the pipeline for treatment of HT</td><td>• Inhibitors of MMP-2 and MMP-9
• Deferoxamine
• Estrogen
• Cilostazol</td></tr>
</table>

Q11. Discuss the management of musculoskeletal pain in patients at risk of renal dysfunction.

Ans. It is estimated that 35–70% of patients with chronic kidney disease (CKD) experience some form of chronic pain and musculoskeletal (MS) pain is the leading cause among them. It is also associated with significant impairment in activities of daily living. MS pain is primarily somatic and can be associated with visceral or neuropathic pain and presents in the form of neck pain, low back pain, joint pain, shoulder girdle pain, muscle catch, etc. Paracetamol (acetaminophen) and nonsteroidal anti-inflammatory drugs (NSAIDs) are commonly used medications for pain management. NSAID use can lead to several adverse effects with gastrointestinal effects and renal dysfunction as a major cause of concern.

In the management of MS pain in patients with impaired renal function or patients at risk of renal derangement, medications with a safe renal profile should be appropriately used. The medications for managing chronic MS pain can be categorized into three main groups—simple analgesics, opioids, and adjuvants **(Table 16)**. It is recommended that step-wise approach, similar to the WHO ladder, is followed in administering medications to these patients, starting with the less potent, safer agents before going for the more potent agents **(Fig. 2)**. Understanding the pharmacokinetic properties of opioids in patients with deranged renal functions is essential before prescribing the right agent **(Table 17)**.

TABLE 16: Medications for management of chronic musculoskeletal pain syndrome.

Simple analgesics			
Paracetamol			
Nonsteroidal anti-inflammatory drug (NSAID) (non-selective)	Aspirin Ibuprofen	Naproxen Aceclofenac	Diclofenac
Selective COX-2 inhibitors	Celecoxib		
Opioids			
Oral	Morphine, methadone, tramadol, and tapentadol		
Intravenous	Morphine, fentanyl, and tramadol		
Transdermal patch	Fentanyl and buprenorphine		
Nasal spray	Tapentadol		
Adjuvants			
Antidepressants	Amitriptyline, nortriptyline, duloxetine, and desvenlafaxine		
Anticonvulsants	Pregabalin, gabapentin, and carbamazepine		
Muscle relaxants	Baclofen, tizanidine, cyclobenzaprine, and tolperisone		
Alpha-2 agonists	Clonidine		
Topical agents			
Capsaicin (0.025–0.075% cream) Diclofenac (1% gel) Ibuprofen (5% cream or gel)	Lidocaine (5%) Ketoprofen (5% cream or gel)	Gabapentin (6% cream or gel) Baclofen (2% cream or gel)	

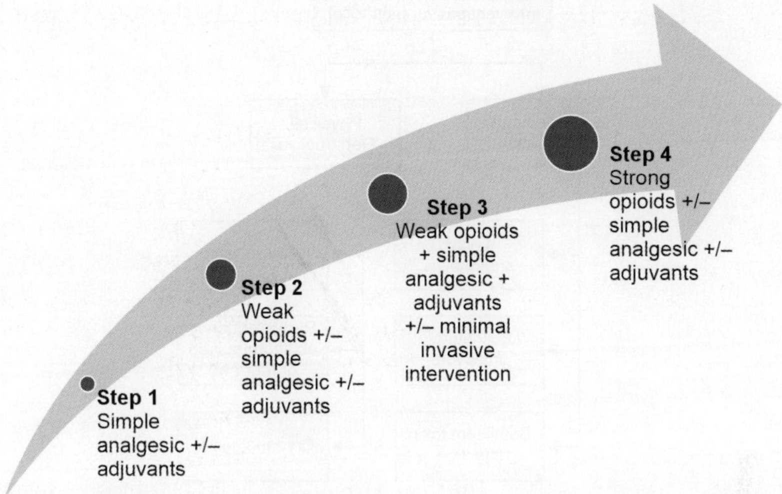

FIG. 2: Ladder approach in pain management.

TABLE 17: Clinical consideration for opioid administration in patients with deranged renal function test (RFT).

Agent	MME conversion factor	Dosing	Adverse effects	Special considerations
Morphine	1	5–15 mg q6–8 h	Nausea, vomiting, sedation, constipation, and respiratory depression	Avoid if CrCl <30 mL/min
Tramadol	0.1	25–50 mg q8–12 h	Headache, sedation, dry mouth, dizziness, and respiratory depression	Maximum dosage is 100 mg BD if CrCl <30 mL/min
Methadone	3	2.5–5 mg q8–12 h	Sedation	No-dose adjustment required in CKD
Fentanyl	0.18	12 mcg/h patch q72 h	Sedation Respiratory depression	TD fentanyl has one of the best safety profiles
Buprenorphine	10	5 µg/h patch every 7 days	Sedation, nausea, vomiting, and headache	TD buprenorphine has one of the best safety profiles
Tapentadol	0.4	50 mg q12 h (maximum dose—500 mg/day)	Nausea, vomiting, constipation, drowsiness, and headache	Avoid if CrCl <30 mL/min
Agents such as meperidine, codeine, and dihydrocodeine are avoided/contraindicated in all stages of CKD.				

[CKD: chronic kidney disease; CrCl: creatinine clearance; MME: morphine milligram equivalent (e.g., tramadol MME 0.1 means 0.1 mg of oral morphine is equipotent to 1 mg of tramadol); TD: transdermal]

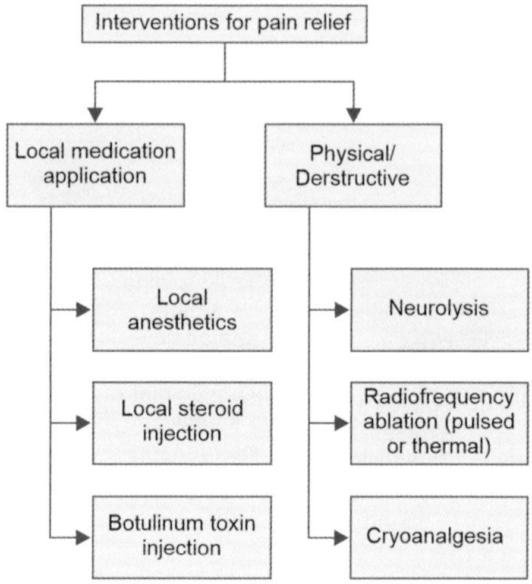

FLOWCHART 10: Interventions to relieve pain in patients with chronic musculoskeletal pain syndromes.

In addition to medications non-pharmacological interventions in the form of cognitive behavior therapy, physical therapy, transcutaneous electrical stimulation, cryotherapy, superficial heat therapy, LASER therapy, acupuncture, passive movements, and range of motion (ROM) exercises have a major supportive role. In patients with refractory pain not responding to medications interventions can be offered. The interventions may be in the form of surgery to address the primary problem leading to the MS pain or minimally invasive procedures to relieve the pain **(Flowchart 10)**.[52-57]

Q12. Management of refractory low back pain with disc prolapse: When and when not to intervene?

Ans. Refractory low back pain is a common clinical scenario. A systematic review of 11 cohort studies by Zhong et al. found that 66% of Lumbar disc herniations have spontaneous resorption.[58] In 2016 New England Journal of Medicine article, Deyo and Mirza recommended surgery for first-time lumbar disc herniation, if there are severe, progressive neurologic deficits with congruent magnetic resonance imaging (MRI) findings and/or if there is failure to conservative treatment after 6 weeks. Bailey et al. reported that microdiscectomy is superior to conservative, non-surgical treatment in reduction of pain intensity at 6 months. The Spine Patient Outcome Research Trial (SPORT) trial demonstrated better outcomes in surgical group in carefully selected patients. Synthesizing the recently published guidelines (23 recommendations since 2011) surgery is recommended when there is a failure of conservative therapy or when progressive/persistent disability is present. Balaji et al. evaluated the role of surgery in patients with motor deficit with MRC grade ≤3 out of 5 and found that surgical intervention is superior. Subsequent studies revealed that preoperative motor strength and time to surgery were the important predictors. Another systematic review showed that preoperative longer symptoms duration adversely impacted postoperative recovery and suggested that "6 months" may represent the cut-off.[59] Younger age, better mental status, and short duration of symptoms predict positive outcomes.

To conclude, the indications for surgery include patients with clinical signs and symptoms associated with lumbar disc herniation, with imaging confirmation of the diagnosis, and lack of improvement after 6 weeks of conservative management. The surgery should not be delayed beyond 6 months. Patients with progressive motor deficit and cauda equina syndrome are also candidates for surgery. Surgery is not indicated in patients with decreased mental status, patients responding to conservative treatment and those with longer duration of symptoms.[59,60]

Q13. How to manage a patient of epilepsy with psychiatric comorbidity?

Ans. Up to 50% of patients with epilepsy develop psychiatric disturbances which can be classified as ictal, inter-ictal and peri-ictal (pre-ictal, post-ictal), and drug related.[61] The prevalence is equal in focal and generalized seizures.[62]

Ictal

They occur for brief period (1–3 minutes) and are associated with ictal phenomenon. Ictal anxiety occurs in up to one-third of patients with focal seizures reporting fear, usually in patients with right temporal foci. Ictal depression is less common. Ictal psychotic symptoms in the form of visual, auditory, and gustatory hallucinations can be associated with focal seizures.

Peri-ictal

Pre-ictal psychiatric disturbances include irritability, depression, aggression, and anxiety. They are relieved by the seizure. They can last for hours to days before the seizure.

Post-ictal confusion is characterized by impaired awareness lasting for few hours. Post-ictal depression can last up to 2 weeks. It occurs more commonly with right-sided temporal or frontal foci. Post-ictal anxiety is less common. Post-ictal psychosis occurs in 6–10% of epilepsy particularly in temporal lobe epilepsy.

Inter-ictal

Depression is present in 40% of patients. Anxiety and bipolar disorders are less common. Interictal psychosis resembles schizophrenia. The risk factors include early age of onset, bilateral temporal foci, a refractory course, and a left-sided epileptic focus.

Treatment-related Psychiatric Problems

Few anti-epileptic drugs can have psychiatric side effects **(Table 18)**. Transient mood disturbances have been reported after temporal lobe surgery for epilepsy.

Management of Psychiatric Disorders in Epilepsy[63]

Depression: Management of psychiatric disorders in epilepsy for depression **(Flowchart 11)**

Anxiety: Management of psychiatric disorders in epilepsy for anxiety **(Flowchart 12)**

Ictal psychosis: Management of psychiatric disorders in epilepsy for ictal psychosis **(Flowchart 13)**

TABLE 18: Psychiatric adverse effects of anti-epileptic medications.

Drug	Psychiatric side effects
Barbiturates	Depression, hyperactivity, irritability, and aggression (especially in children)
Benzodiazepines	Hyperactivity, irritability, and aggression in children and elderly
Levetiracetam	Depression, psychosis, and suicidal thoughts
Ampanel	Depression and suicidal thoughts
Ethosuximide	Psychosis
Felbamate	Anxiety and psychosis
Lamotrigine	Hyperactivity, irritability, and aggression in children
Vigabatrin	Depression
Zonisamide	Psychosis, depression, and irritability

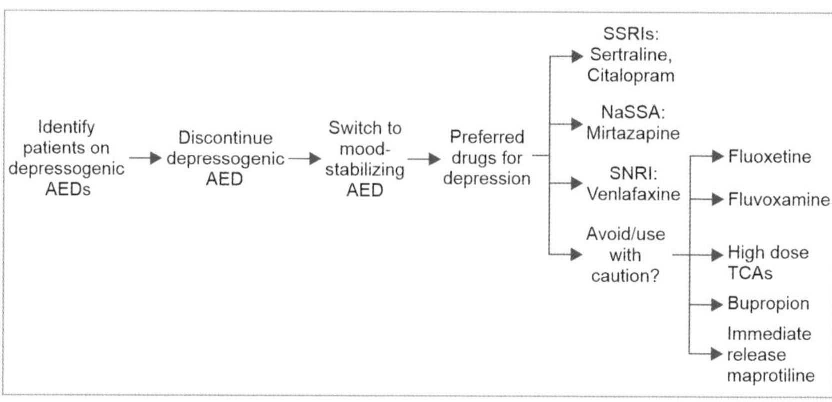

FLOWCHART 11: Management of psychiatric disorders in epilepsy for depression.

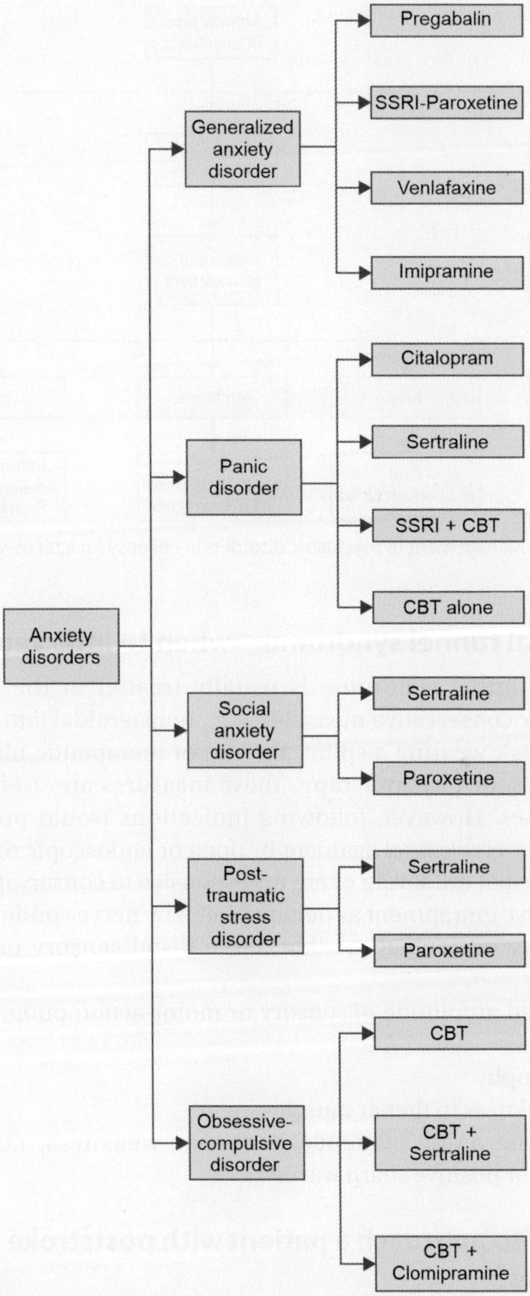

FLOWCHART 12: Management of psychiatric disorders in epilepsy for anxiety

(CBT: cognitive behavioral therapy)

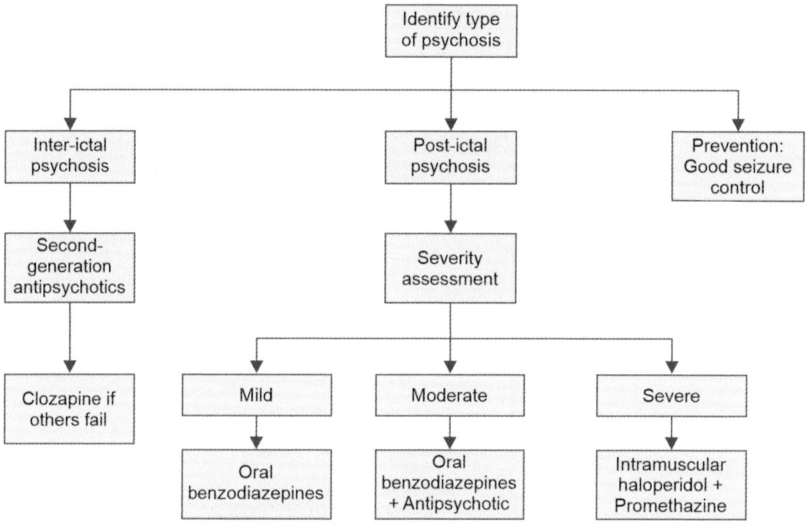

FLOWCHART 13: Management of psychiatric disorders in epilepsy for ictal psychosis.

Q14. Carpal tunnel syndrome—when to intervene?

Ans. Carpal tunnel syndrome is usually treated in the beginning by nonsurgical or conservative measures, e.g., nonsteroidal anti-inflammatory drugs (NSAIDs), wearing a splint, the use of therapeutic ultrasound, oral corticosteroids, or physiotherapy. These measures are useful in mild-to-moderate cases. However, following indications would prompt surgical release of transverse carpal ligament by open or endoscopic routes:

- Symptoms that are severe or are unresponsive to conservative measures.
- Severe nerve entrapment as demonstrated by nerve conduction studies:
    - Severely prolonged median nerve distal sensory or distal motor latency
    - Reduced amplitude of sensory or motor action potential in median nerve
- Thenar atrophy
- Motor weakness in thenar muscles
- Electromyographic evidence of thenar weakness, i.e., fibrillation potentials or positive sharp waves[64]

Q15. How to approach a patient with poststroke swallowing issues?

Ans. Stroke can result in swallowing issues or dysphagia due to damage anywhere along the deglutitive axis, which are as follow:

- *Brain*:
    - Lateral motor cortex within the inferior precentral gyrus (area of cortical representation for tongue and face)
    - Supplementary motor cortex
    - Anterior cingulate gyrus
    - Insula
    - Cerebellum
- *Brainstem*:
    - Central pattern generators within the reticular formation direct the sequential movements of various muscles involved in swallowing
    - Motor nuclei—nucleus ambiguous and the dorsal motor nucleus of vagus directly control motor output to the pharyngeal muscle and proximal esophagus
    - Sensory nuclei—nucleus tractus solitarius and spinal nucleus of trigeminal system
- *Nerves:* Five cranial nerves (V, VII, IX, X, and XII)
- *Muscles:* Oropharyngeal, laryngeal, and esophageal muscles

Dysphagia can have serious consequences such as aspiration pneumonia, malnutrition, and dehydration. Hence, thorough assessment of poststroke dysphagia is necessary. When dysphagia is suspected, patient to be kept nil per mouth and swallow screening, e.g., with Gugging Swallowing Screen (GUSS) **(Table 19)** is to be done within 24 hours. Once screening is positive, thorough evaluation to be done.

Good history can provide useful clues to possible neuromuscular disorder in different phases **(Table 20)**.

Next, clinically assess the following:

- Inspect the oral cavity—look for any obvious pathology, e.g., enlarged tonsils, adenoids, candidiasis, etc.
- Examination of V, VII, IX, X, and XIIth cranial nerves
- Pseudobulbar signs
- Dyskinesia of face, jaw, or tongue

Associated clinical findings will guide you to localize the lesion and identify the etiopathology, e.g., history of (h/o) diurnal variation in neuromuscular junction disorder, generalized hyporeflexia in cranial neuropathy due to acute inflammatory demyelinating polyneuropathy (AIDP), and long tract signs in brainstem lesions.

Finally, swallowing can be instrumentally evaluated using videofluoroscopic swallowing study (gold standard method that assesses diet consistency, delay in start of swallowing, and oral transit time), functional endoscopic evaluation of swallow, swallowing ultrasound, swallowing surface electromyography, and laryngoscopy (mirror or fiberoptic).[65]

TABLE 19: Gugging Swallowing Screen (GUSS).

<table>
<tr><td colspan="4">1. Preliminary investigation/indirect swallowing test:</td></tr>
<tr><td></td><td>YES</td><td colspan="2">NO</td></tr>
<tr><td>Vigilance (The patient must be alert for at least 15 minutes)</td><td>1 ☐</td><td colspan="2">0 ☐</td></tr>
<tr><td>Cough and/or throat clearing (Voluntary cough! Patient should cough or clear his or her throat twice)</td><td>1 ☐</td><td colspan="2">0 ☐</td></tr>
<tr><td>Saliva swallow
Swallowing successful</td><td>1 ☐</td><td colspan="2">0 ☐</td></tr>
<tr><td>Drooling (Herausrinnen von Speichel aus dem Mund)</td><td>0 ☐</td><td colspan="2">1 ☐</td></tr>
<tr><td>Voice change (hoarse, gurgely, coated, weak, choke on own saliva)</td><td>0 ☐</td><td colspan="2">1 ☐</td></tr>
<tr><td>SUM:</td><td colspan="3">(5)</td></tr>
<tr><td></td><td colspan="3">1 – 4 = Investigate further
5 = Continue with "direct swallowing test"</td></tr>
<tr><td colspan="4">2. Direct swallowing test:
(Material: Aqua bi, flat teaspoon, food thickener, and bread)</td></tr>
<tr><td>In the following order:</td><td>1 →</td><td>2 →</td><td>3 →</td></tr>
<tr><td></td><td>Semisolid</td><td>Liquid</td><td>Solid</td></tr>
<tr><td>Deglutition:</td><td></td><td></td><td></td></tr>
<tr><td>Swallowing not possible</td><td>0 ☐</td><td>0 ☐</td><td>0 ☐</td></tr>
<tr><td>Swallowing delayed (>2 seconds)
(Solid textures >10 seconds)</td><td>1 ☐</td><td>1 ☐</td><td>1 ☐</td></tr>
<tr><td>Swallowing successful</td><td>2 ☐</td><td>2 ☐</td><td>2 ☐</td></tr>
<tr><td colspan="4">Cough (involuntary):
(before, during, or after swallowing—until 3 minutes later)</td></tr>
<tr><td>Yes</td><td>0 ☐</td><td>0 ☐</td><td>0 ☐</td></tr>
<tr><td>No</td><td>1 ☐</td><td>1 ☐</td><td>1 ☐</td></tr>
<tr><td colspan="4">Drooling:</td></tr>
<tr><td>Yes</td><td>0 ☐</td><td>0 ☐</td><td>0 ☐</td></tr>
<tr><td>No</td><td>1 ☐</td><td>1 ☐</td><td>1 ☐</td></tr>
<tr><td colspan="4">Voice change:
(listen to the voice before and after swallowing – patient should speak "oh")</td></tr>
<tr><td>Yes</td><td>0 ☐</td><td>0 ☐</td><td>0 ☐</td></tr>
<tr><td>No</td><td>1 ☐</td><td>1 ☐</td><td>1 ☐</td></tr>
<tr><td>SUM:</td><td>(5)</td><td>(5)</td><td>(5)</td></tr>
<tr><td></td><td>1–4 investigate further
5 = Continue "Liquid"</td><td>1–4 investigate further
5 = Continue "Solid"</td><td>1–4 investigate further
5 = "Normal"</td></tr>
</table>

TABLE 20: Symptoms of swallowing dysfunction at different stages.

Oral phase	Pharyngeal phase	Esophageal phase
• Drooling in nonmeal time • Food spillage and cannot take food from utensils • Cannot use straw • Inability to chew • Difficulty to initiate swallowing	• Food gets stuck at base of tongue or bottom of throat immediately after swallowing • History of repeated attempts for successful swallowing • History of cough or choking before, during, or after swallowing • History of nasal regurgitation and wet voice following ingestion of liquids	• Onset of symptoms several seconds after initiation of swallowing • Sensation of food hanging up in the suprasternal notch or retrosternal area

Q16. How to approach a patient with poststroke speech and language issues?

Ans. Aphasia is observed with a prevalence ranging from 16 to 45% in stroke patients, most studies converging to 30% at admission and 18% at discharge.[66] Aphasia is a marker of stroke severity and is associated with higher risk of mortality,[67] poor functional prognosis,[68] and increased risk of poststroke dementia.[69]

The approach to language disturbances is clinically based on oral production and comprehension.

Assessment of oral production examines *fluency* (nonfluent aphasia/ expressive one being characterized by less than seven words in utterances. This is associated with difficulty in initiation and/or agrammatism. There are deviations at various levels such as articulation level (articulatory defect), phonemic (omission, substitution, addition, or inversion of phoneme), verbal (ventral paraphasia, word-finding difficulty, circumlocution, perseveration, and neologism), syntactic (agrammatism characterized by omission of articles, preposition, auxiliary verbs, and inflexions leading to telegraphic speech).

Fluent aphasia/receptive one is characterized by increased fluency associated with phonemic and verbal deviations leading to jargonaphasia and neologism. *Comprehension* at the level of word and syntax is impaired. When to suspect? A patient does not behave according to the examiner's instruction during examination. Object pointing on verbal command and instructions based on sentences of gradual complexities are impaired.

Aphasic syndromes are classified by testing fluency, comprehension, naming, repetition, reading, and writing. 10% of aphasic patients are not classifiable, particularly in recurrent stroke **(Table 21)**.[66-69]

TABLE 21: Types of aphasia.

	Comprehension	Repetition of spoken language	Naming	Fluency
Wernicke's	Impaired	Impaired	Impaired	Preserved or increased
Broca's	Preserved (except grammar)	Impaired	Impaired	Decreased
Global	Impaired	Impaired	Impaired	Decreased
Conduction	Preserved	Preserved	Impaired	Preserved
Nonfluent (anterior) transcortical	Preserved	Preserved	Impaired	Impaired
Fluent (posterior) transcortical	Impaired	Preserved	Impaired	Preserved
Isolation	Impaired	Echolalia	Impaired	No purposeful speech
Anomic	Preserved	Preserved	Impaired	Preserved except for word-finding pauses
Pure word deafness	Impaired only for spoken language	Impaired	Preserved	Preserved
Pure alexia	Impaired only for reading	Preserved	Preserved	Preserved

Q17. How to select the ideal agent for secondary stroke prevention?

Ans. For secondary stroke prevention, different strategies can be applied which include lifestyle modification (diet changes, reduction of salt intake, exercise, abstinence from smoking); medical management (antihypertensive therapy, antithrombotic therapy with antiplatelet agents or anticoagulants, lipid-lowering therapy and agents for glycemic control) and procedural interventions (carotid endarterectomy or stenting). The present discussion will be restricted to the medical management for secondary stroke prevention.

- *Antihypertensive therapy*:
  - In patients with stroke or transient ischemic attack or nondiabetic chronic kidney disease and stroke, antihypertensive treatment must aim to achieve a target of consistently lower than 140/90 mm Hg.
  - In patients with small subcortical stroke, target systolic blood pressure should be lowerthan130 mm Hg.

  - For patients with diabetes, target systolic and diastolic blood pressures must be lower than 130 and 80 mm Hg respectively.
  - As per available evidence, diuretic or a combination of diuretic with angiotensin-converting enzyme inhibitor is most suitable. However, concomitant clinical conditions, long-term tolerance to the drug and extent of reduction of hypertension would govern the final choice of antihypertensive agent.
- *Antiplatelet therapy*:
  - With the exception of cardioembolic stroke, for majority of stroke subtypes, antiplatelet agents are the antithrombotic agents of choice for secondary stroke prevention.
  - The available options are Aspirin (81–325 mg daily), Clopidogrel (75 mg daily), combination of extended-release aspirin and dipyridamole.
  - A reasonable approach would be to administer dual antiplatelet therapy with aspirin and clopidogrel for 21 days followed by a single antiplatelet therapy thereafter.
  - Chronic administration of combined clopidogrel and aspirin is not recommended for secondary stroke prevention, unless there is an alternate indication (e.g., coronary drug-eluting stent requiring dual antiplatelet therapy).
- *Anticoagulation therapy*:
  - Anticoagulation is justified for cardioembolic stroke including nonvalvular atrial fibrillation, known left atrial or left ventricular thrombus, mechanical left ventricular assist device, left ventricular ejection fraction less than 35% and valvular heart disease.
  - Compared to warfarin, direct oral anticoagulants (e.g., dabigatran, direct thrombin inhibitor as well as rivaroxaban, apixaban and edoxaban) have similar efficacy for prevention of thromboembolic events and lower risk of intracranial haemorrhage. But, direct oral anticoagulants are not safe in renal impairment.
  - For patients with mechanical heart valves, warfarin is recommended.
- *Lipid-lowering therapy*:
  - The first-line agent for dyslipidemia after stroke is statins. In case of intolerance or inadequate response to statins, ezetimibe may be considered.
  - Target is to achieve a level of LDL cholesterol consistently less than 2.0 mmol/L or >50% reduction from baseline. If stroke is associated with concomitant acute coronary syndrome or established coronary disease, LDL must be more aggressively reduced to less than 1.8 mmol/L or > 50% reduction.
- *Glycemic control*: Although individualisation is required, reduction of HbA1c levels to 7% in both type 1 and type 2 diabetes would be prudent. Even though pioglitazone has demonstrated benefits for secondary stroke prevention in patients with insulin resistance, its use is restricted by its adverse events.[70,71]

Q18. When to suspect secondary headache?

Ans. Secondary headaches are those in which the headache is a symptom of an underlying medical condition. The various causes of secondary headache include:

- Vascular (e.g., subarachnoid hemorrhage, cerebral venous thrombosis, temporal arteritis, and pituitary apoplexy)
- Infections (e.g., meningitis, brain abscess, and encephalitis)
- Toxins and drugs (e.g., inhalation of carbon monoxide, ingestion of nitrates and nitrites, misuse of analgesics, substance abuse, and withdrawal of drugs)
- Brain tumors
- Benign intracranial hypertension
- Ophthalmological (e.g., glaucoma)
- Endocrine and metabolic (e.g., pheochromocytoma, hypoxia, and hypercapnia)
- Miscellaneous (e.g., postdural puncture headache and hypertension)

The *SNOOP* mnemonic can be an useful adjunct to help us identify secondary headaches. The indicators are:

- *S*: Systemic symptoms and signs: History of malignancy, immunosuppression, fever, and night sweats
- *N*: Neurologic symptoms and signs: Focal or global neurological deficit including loss of consciousness, behavioral alterations, motor weakness, sensory loss, ataxia, diplopia, or transient visual blurring
- *O*: Onset—sudden onset that is reaches peak within 1 minute, also known as thunderclap headache
- *O*: Onset age—new onset headache in age <5 years or >65 years
- *P*:
    - *Pattern change*: Evolution to daily headache or change in headache characteristics
    - Precipitated by Valsalva maneuver
    - Postural aggravation
    - Papilledema
    - Pulsatile tinnitus
    - *Pregnancy*: New onset headache during pregnancy
    - Phenotype of rare variety, e.g., hypnic, cough-, sex- or exercise-induced[72]

Q19. What are the medications for stroke rehabilitation—rationale for administration?

Ans. Till date, the search for a 'miracurol' or 'magic pill' to treat motor deficits after stroke has yielded futile results. Although agents like dopamine agonists like amphetamine and levodopa, acetylcholinesterase inhibitor donepezil and SSRI fluoxetine initially demonstrated promising results, large randomised clinical trials ultimately dispelled the optimism.

However, medicines are necessary to treat the following conditions, which otherwise would impede the process of rehabilitation and recovery in stroke patients:

- *Spasticity*: Oral agents, e.g., baclofen, clonazepam and parenteral botulinum injections might help.
- *Pain*: Stroke may result in both nociceptive pain as well as neuropathic pain. Nociceptive pain may be treated by physiotherapy and NSAIDs, whereas, neuropathic pain may be managed by gabapentin and pregabalin.
- *Deep vein thrombosis and pulmonary embolism*: These emergency conditions require prompt intervention. Low-molecular weight heparin and compression stockings are to be administered.
- *Pressure ulcers, urinary and fecal incontinence and aspiration pneumonia*: Depending on patient profile, physicians must institute antibiotics as may be appropriate.[73,74]

Q20. What are the evaluation and management of erectile dysfunction?

Ans. Erectile dysfunction (ED) can be defined as "persistent inability to develop and maintain an erection sufficient for satisfactory sexual activity." Detailed history and clinical examination may help to identify the site of lesion.

- *Temporal lobe and hypothalamic disease*: Loss of desire
- *Spinal cord disease*:
  - *Spinal cord lesion in cervical or high thoracic lesions*:
    - Preserved reflex erections, but unable to sustain erection for penetrative intercourse
    - Ejaculation and orgasm may be affected.
  - *Spinal cord lesion in S2-S4*: Loss of reflex erection but psychogenic erection possible
- *Cauda equina lesions*:
  - Reflex erection lost
  - Somatic sensation in S2-S4 dermatomes is impaired.
  - In situations where only pelvic nerves are damaged but pudendal nerves are spared. ED occurs with preserved somatic sensation.
- *Small fiber neuropathy*: ED may occur early without disturbance of ejaculation or bladder dysfunction.

Lifestyle modification, e.g., reducing alcohol intake, weight reduction, and smoking cessation are the initial measures in managing ED. The current management strategies for treatment of ED include oral phosphodiesterase-5 inhibitors (e.g., tadalafil and sildenafil), intracavernous injection (with papaverine, prostaglandin E1, and phentolamine), vacuum erection device, low intensity extracorporeal shockwave, and penile prosthesis implantation.[65,75]

Q21. Discuss the approach to unilateral drooping of eye lid.

Ans. Drooping of eyelid or ptosis can be due to a weakness in levator palpebrae superioris (LPS) or Müller's muscle (oculosympathetic pathway). If due to LPS weakness, the ptosis is complete, incorrectable, and associated with extraocular muscle (EOM) weakness and pupillary dilation. On the other hand, ptosis resultant from Müller's palsy is incomplete, correctable, with dilated pupils, but no EOM weakness.

If LPS is the culprit muscle, localize the lesion at the following levels according to **Table 22**:

- Muscle
- Neuromuscular junction
- Third cranial nerve

Very rarely, a unilateral cerebral hemispheric lesion (e.g., due to stroke) may cause contralateral or bilateral ptosis.

Whereas ptosis due to Müller's muscle palsy can be a result of lesion at the following anatomical substrates:

- First order neuron (central, i.e., hypothalamus, brainstem, and spinal cord) due to stroke, demyelination, tumor, and syringomyelia
- Second order neuron (preganglionic) due to brachial plexus lesion, apical lung tumor, thoracic surgery, jugular or subclavian artery injury, insertion of chest tubes, or central lines
- Third order neuron (postganglionic, i.e., superior cervical ganglion, internal carotid artery, skull base, and cavernous sinus) due to internal carotid artery dissection or aneurysm, cavernous sinus thrombosis, and nasopharyngeal carcinoma[65]

Q22. Discuss the approach to walking and leaking patient.

Ans. By the term leaking patient, we essentially mean here bladder dysfunction. When a physician wishes to analyze symptoms of bladder dysfunction, he/she must first determine whether it is due to neurological illness or mechanical problem in bladder outlet. Once ascertained as a neurological problem, detailed history taking and clinical examination can help determine the site of lesion.

- Is it due to a neurological disorder?
  Abnormal neurological examination and a combination of blader symptoms, ED, constipation, and fecal incontinence strongly hint toward a neurological origin[65]
- Is it UMN bladder or LMN bladder? **(Table 23)**
- Localize the lesion **(Table 24)**

Q23. What is the approach to tinnitus?

Ans. Tinnitus, a sensation of hearing noise in absence of any external or internal source, is often described by patients as ringing, humming, or whistling sound. Although mostly idiopathic and benign, it can stem from multiple causes. Targeted history, physical examination, and audiological

TABLE 22: Causes and localization of ptosis due to LPS palsy.

Site of lesion	Common causes	Localizing clinical findings
Muscle	• Aponeurotic defect (levator dehiscence) due to aging, trauma, and ocular surgery • Chronic progressive external ophthalmoplegia (CPEO) • Myotonic dystrophy • Oculopharyngeal muscular dystrophy	
Neuromuscular junction	Myasthenia gravis	• Diurnal variation • Subacute onset, gradually progressive
	Snake bite	History of a bite
	Botulism	History of ingestion of canned food and diarrhea. Examination may reveal descending flaccid paralysis.
Third cranial nerve		
Nucleus	• Complete, ipsilateral third nerve palsy • Bilateral ptosis (as both LPS are innervated by single, midline LPS subnucleus) • Contralateral superior rectus palsy	Stroke Demyelination Tumor Infection (e.g., NCC and TB)
Fascicle	• Usually, accompanied by other neurological findings: • Contralateral hemiparesis due to cerebral peduncle lesion • Contralateral tremors due to red nucleus involvement • Medial lemniscus involvement	Same as in nucleus
Subarachnoid space	• Pupillary involvement is common due to superficial, dorsomedial location of pupillary fibers at this level. • May present with headache/orbital pain/meningeal signs	• ICA/PCOM/PCA/basilar artery aneurysm • Meningitis • Trauma (head injury) • Uncal herniation
Cavernous sinus	Concurrent features of IVth, VIth, V1 involvement	• Cavernous sinus thrombosis • Carotid aneurysm • Caroticocavernous fistula • Neoplasm
Orbital apex	• Features of IInd nerve involvement along with IVth, VIth, and V1 cranial nerves • Proptosis and conjunctival chemosis	Trauma Neoplasm Infection (fungus)

(ICA: internal carotid artery; LPS: levator palpebrae superioris; NCC: neurocysticercosis; PCA: posterior cerebral artery; PCOM: posterior communicating artery; TB: tuberculosis)

TABLE 23: Differences between UMN bladder and LMN bladder.

UMN bladder (i.e., above conus medullaris and cauda equina)	LMN bladder (i.e., at conus medullaris, cauda equina, and S2-S4 segments of spinal cord)
Clues: • Increased frequency • Urgency, urge incontinence • Voluntary control—lost • Residual urine volume—increased • Bulbocavernosus and anal reflex—present	*Clues*: • Overdistended bladder • Residual urine volume is more than in UMN bladder. • Retention of urine • Overflow incontinence • Stress incontinence • Saddle anesthesia • Loss of bulbocavernosus and anal reflex

(LMN: lower motor neuron; UMN: upper motor neuron)

TABLE 24: Localization of lesion in bladder dysfunction.

Location	Clinical clues	Etiology
UMN		
Suprapontine	• Loss of voluntary control of micturition • Bladder sensation is normal • Postvoid residual urine volume not increased	• Frontal lobe space occupying lesion • Normal pressure hydrocephalus • Stroke • Dementia
Spinal		
Spinal shock	Overflow incontinence	Acute transverse myelopathy
Reflex neurogenic bladder/ spastic bladder	• Detrusor sphincter dyssynergia present • Initiation of voluntary micturition impaired • Bladder capacity is reduced but residual urine volume is raised.	• Slowly evolving lesion in cord • Recovery from spinal shock • Partial lesion of cord
LMN		
Conus medullaris/ cauda equina	• Impaired sensation of bladder fullness • Voluntary control of micturition lost • Overflow incontinence • Large residual urine volume and urinary tract infection	• Spinal cord injury • Necrotizing myelitis • Spinal cord tumor
Motor paralytic bladder	• Painful urinary retention • Overflow incontinence—large residual volume	• Pelvic trauma • Major pelvic surgery • Disk herniation • Guillain–Barré syndrome • Lower spinal cord tumor
Sensory paralytic bladder	• Painless urinary retention • Overflow incontinence • Patients able to void voluntarily	• Tabes dorsalis • Diabetes mellitus • Syringomyelia

(LMN: lower motor neuron; UMN: upper motor neuron)

TABLE 25: Etiologies of tinnitus.

Tonal tinnitus	Nontonal tinnitus

Signifies a disorder of auditory conduction and transduction pathway:
• External ear: Cerumen impaction
• Middle ear:
  ○ Otitis media
  ○ Mastoiditis
• Inner ear:
  ○ Meniere's disease
  ○ Vestibular schwannoma
  ○ Otosclerosis
  ○ Labyrinthitis
  ○ Presbyacusis
  ○ Noise exposure
  ○ Ototoxicity/vestibulotoxicity (antibiotics, analgesics, chemotherapeutic agents, corticosteroids, diuretics, and NSAIDs)
	• Contraction of muscles of eustachian tube, tympanic cavity (stapedius and tensor tympani), palate (palatal myoclonus), and pharynx
	• Pulsatile tinnitus:
	  ○ Raised intracranial tension due to any cause, whereby, venous turbulence on account of pressure gradient between cranial and cervical venous structures contributes to the noise
	  ○ Vascular ear tumors (e.g., glomus tympanicum and glomus jugulare)
	  ○ Arterial bruit
	  ○ Venous hum
	  ○ Arteriovenous malformation
	  ○ Intracranial aneurysm
	  ○ Vascular tumors of skull such as histiocytosis X

(NSAIDs: nonsteroidal anti-inflammatory drugs)

evaluation must be conducted to rule out ominous causes such as vascular tumors or vestibular schwannoma.

Tinnitus can be tonal or nontonal. The more common type, tonal is also called "subjective" as it can be perceived only by the patient. Whereas nontonal type is sometimes referred to as "objective" as it can be heard by both patient and examiner. Different causes of tinnitus have been enumerated in **Table 25**.

Important clinical findings and their interpretations have been summarized in **Table 26**.[65,76-78]

Q24. Discuss the approach to a patient with recurrent falls.

Ans. At the outset, it is important to distinguish whether you are dealing with a case of drop attack or falls. Drop attack usually means a sudden fall without a prodrome that may or may not be accompanied by loss of consciousness. Drop attacks could be due to syncope, seizures, transient ischemic attacks, third ventricular and posterior fossa tumors, otolithic crisis (e.g., Tumarkin's phenomenon in Meneire's disease) or cataplexy. On the other hand, falls represent incapability to remain upright due to lesion in any of the structures responsible for maintenance of normal posture, stance, and gait. Those structures responsible for a normal gait cycle have been enumerated in **Flowchart 14**. At least two such falls in a 12-month period are defined as recurrent falls. Besides, recurrent falls are common in elderly due to their growing infirmities. In fact, the very fear of falling, in itself, aggravates the risk

TABLE 26: Clinical findings and interpretations in tinnitus.

Finding	Interpretation
History	
Location	If unilateral, more likely to be a focal lesion, e.g., vestibular schwannoma or vascular tumor
Duration	If acute (<6 months), probably due to noise trauma, ototoxicity, and otitis media. Chronic tinnitus (>6 months) is less likely to resolve spontaneously.
Character	• Low frequency or "whooshing" or blowing may be due to conductive hearing loss. • High frequency or "chirping" may be because of sensorineural hearing loss. • Rhythmic clicking due to palatal or middle ear myoclonus
Associated findings	• *Ear drainage or ear pain*: Consider infectious etiology • *Vertigo and imbalance*: Consider cochlear, retrocochlear, or central nervous system (CNS) lesions (e.g., Meniere's disease and vestibular schwannoma)
Precipitating factors	Tinnitus on change in head position may indicate raised intracranial tension.
Examination	
Ear	Detailed examination to find out the etiology
Eye	Papilledema indicates intracranial hypertension
Muscular	Temporomandibular joint (TMJ) tenderness suggestive of TMJ disorders
Neurologic	Gaze-evoked nystagmus may occur following removal of cerebellopontine angle tumors. Abnormal VIIIth nerve findings may suggest vestibular schwannoma.
Vascular	Bruit over the mastoid process suggests vascular tumor or arteriovenous malformation Obliteration of tinnitus on pressing jugular vein suggests venous origin

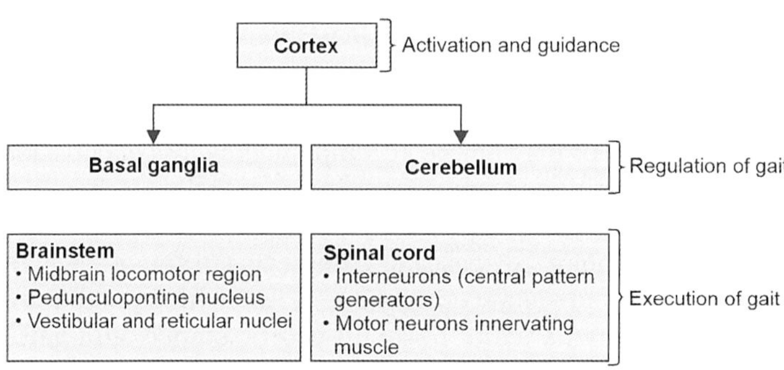

FLOWCHART 14: Neural control of gait.

of falling and subsequent immobilization. Also, myriad of other conditions, e.g., polypharmacy with different psychoactive drugs, cardiovascular drugs (e.g., diuretics and antiarrhythmics), anticholinergic drugs; skeletal deformities, e.g., osteoarthritis; metabolic disorders (e.g., hyponatremia), and cognitive decline may also contribute to recurrent falls.

First, elicit a detailed history from the patient. Important clinical clues may be revealed as follows:

- *Onset and progression*: For example, in idiopathic parkinson disease (IPD), gait disorder progresses very slowly, and falls occur in the later part of the disease, whereas in progressive supranuclear palsy (PSP), there is rapid worsening of gait with frequent falls early in the course of the disease.
- History of falls:
    - Ask whether it was an unprotected fall (fall like a log of wood) with multiple injuries which is more common in gait disorders associated with loss of postural reflexes. Always rule out other causes of fall, e.g., syncope, epileptic drop attacks, vertebrobasilar transient ischemic attack, and cataplexy.
    - PSP patient falls even when standing, IPD patient falls while turning or changing posture.
    - Nonpatterned fall occurs in dementia due to lack of attention and insight leading to carelessness.
    - Fall with bizarre acrobatic posture (patient usually lands safely) occurs in functional gait disorder.
- *History of diurnal variation:*
    - Sensory ataxia increases in darkness
    - Gait difficulty increases as the day progresses in dopa responsive dystonia
        - *Difficulties in going up the stairs:* Hip extensor weakness
        - *Difficulties in going down the stairs:* Quadriceps weakness
- *Tripping or stumbling of feet:* Due to foot drop, spasticity, shallow steps of basal ganglia disorder, or frontal lobe gait.
- History of joint pain and swelling
- History of neurogenic claudication
- Drug history

Next, go for physical examination (look for joint pain/swelling, range of joint movement, skeletal deformity, and spine deformity), neurological examination (assessment of cognitive function, motor, sensory, cerebellar systems, and postural reflexes), and gait examination.

Majorly, recurrent falls are either due to ataxia or gait disorders. Their principal types and clinical clues have been enlisted in **Tables 27 and 28**, respectively.[65,79,80]

TABLE 27: Localization of ataxia.

Anatomical substrate	Clinical clues	Examination clues	Further localization		
Cerebellar	• Gait ataxia • Truncal ataxia • Limb ataxia • Tremulousness of limbs • Slurring of speech	• Intention tremor • Finger nose test • Rebound phenomenon • Dysdiadochokinesia • Impaired tandem walking • Hypotonia • Scanning speech • Oculomotor abnormalities	Zone	Clinical manifestations	
			Medial	Nystagmus, oculomotor disturbances, and gait ataxia	
			Intermediate	Gait and stance ataxia, dysarthria	
			Lateral	Limb ataxia	
			Pancerebellar	All of the above	
Sensory	• Sensory symptoms, e.g., paresthesias and numbness • Band-like sensation, plaster cast sensation • Disproportionate aggravation of symptoms in darkness • Normal speech	• Impaired vibration and position sense • Deep tendon reflexes may be lost. • No oculomotor disturbance • High steppage gait	Site	Symptom	Sign
			Peripheral nerve (large fiber)	Glove and stocking distribution	Lower motor neuron (LMN) signs
			Dorsal root ganglion	Nonlength-dependent symptoms	Sensory motor dissociation
			Posterior column in spinal cord	Definite sensory levels	Signs of myelopathy
			Medial lemniscus in brainstem	Brainstem symptoms	Brainstem signs
			Parietal lobe	Seizures, and headache	Impairment of cortical sensation
Vestibular	• Presence of prominent vertigo • Speech is relatively spared • Nausea and vomiting • Tinnitus, deafness, and aural fullness	• Head impulse test is positive. • Characteristic peripheral vestibular nystagmus • Vestibuloocular reflex deranged			

TABLE 28: Summary of gait disorders.

Gait disorder	Gait initiation	Step length	Step height	Cadence	Base	Others
High level	Hesitancy	Short	Short	Lower	Wide	• Magnetic gait
Spastic	–	Short	Short	Regular	Wide	• Circumduction • Scissoring
Extra-pyramidal	–	Short	Short	Low	Narrow	• ↓ arm swing • Festination • Freezing • Turns en bloc
Cerebellar	–	Variable	Variable	Irregular	Wide	• Tandem gait impaired
Sensory ataxia	–	Short	↑	–	Wide	• Thumping gait • Diurnal variation

Q25. What is approach to a patient with double vision?

Ans. Misalignment of the eyes due to any deviation from normal eye movement is perceived as double vision (diplopia). The following stepwise approach would help you to diagnose the cause of diplopia:

1. Step I: Is it monocular or binocular diplopia?
    - Once diplopia resolves on closing either eye, it is monocular diplopia. It can be because of a refractive problem (e.g., astigmatism) or an ocular disease (e.g., corneal pathology, cataract, and severe retinal pathology)
    - However, if the diplopia is persistent in spite of closing either eye, it is binocular diplopia. In this case, you need to answer thee questions:
        i. Which eye muscles are weak?
        ii. Where is the lesion—supranuclear, internuclear, nuclear/infranuclear, muscles, or orbital tissue?
        iii. What is the likely etiopathology?
2. *Step II: History—key questions*:
    a. How are the two images separated—horizontally, vertically, or obliquely?
        - Horizontal diplopia—medial rectus or lateral rectus palsy
        - *Vertical diplopia*:
            - Impaired elevation or depression
            - Usually seen in superior oblique palsy or skew deviation. In superior oblique palsy, diplopia is vertical and torsional (lower image is tilted). But in skew deviation (brainstem or cerebellar pathology), diplopia is purely vertical.
        - *Oblique diplopia*: Oculomotor palsies (since both vertical and horizontal motility are affected)

TABLE 29: Worsening of double vision in different gazes.	
Direction of worsening	**Weakness**
Lateral gaze in one direction	Ipsilateral lateral rectus or contralateral medial rectus
Upgaze	Inferior oblique or superior rectus
Downgaze	Superior oblique or inferior rectus
Comitant (does not change with direction of gaze)	Congenital strabismus, skew deviation

b. Is double vision worse at distance or at near?
   - Worsening at distance (e.g., during driving)—lateral rectus weakness (abduction is required for divergence)
   - Worsening at near (e.g., during reading)—medical rectus weakness (adduction is required for convergence)

c. *Does the double vision worsen (i.e., distance between two images increase) in a particular gaze?* ***(Table 29)***

d. *Is there any h/o abnormal head posture?*
   The patient assumes a head position to turn the eyes away from the field of action of the weak muscle. Hence if head is flexed, superior rectus is weak; if extended, inferior rectus is weak, and if tilted toward the shoulder on one side, contralateral superior oblique is weak.

e. *Is double vision intermittent or constant?*
   Double vision only on certain tasks, in some specific environment or after fatigue is called intermittent diplopia. Diplopia worsening with fatigue suggests myasthenia gravis or decompensation of a longstanding strabismus.

f. *Is there any h/o childhood orthoptic treatment or h/o of recent/remote head trauma?*
   Such diplopia is usually due to decompensation of a longstanding phoria which was normalized by fusional mechanism.

g. *What are the other neurological symptoms?*
   Help to identify site of lesion and underlying cause.
   - H/o headache—aneurysmal third nerve palsy and diabetic cranial neuropathy (microvascular)
   - H/o diminished visual acuity—localizes lesion in orbital apex

3. Step III: Examine –
   - Eyelid—check for ptosis
   - Eye movements—examine following eye movements:
     - *Fixation (gaze holding)*: Check for any instability of fixation(e.g., square wave jerks, and nystagmus)
     - Monocular eye movement (duction)
     - Binocular eye movements (version)
     - Convergence and divergence
     - Saccades and pursuit in both horizontal and vertical planes
   - Forced duction test
   - Vestibulocular reflex—head thrust test

- Look for nystagmus and other ocular oscillations
- Light and accommodation reflex
- Visual acuity and ophthalmoscopy
- General neurologic examination for localization and diagnosis of primary neurological disorder[65]

Q26. What is the approach to a patient with acute onset unilateral loss of vision?

Ans. Acute onset unilateral loss of vision may be due to a lesion in the eye itself or in the visual pathway anterior to chiasma. The localizing clinical features and possible etiologies have been given here:

- *Ocular media (cornea, aqueous humor, lens, vitreous humor, choroid)*:
    - H/o eye pain, redness of eye, and watering from eyes
    - May improve with glasses
    - Pinhole test—may be positive
    - Red reflex—may be abnormal
    - No relative afferent pupillary defect (RAPD)
    - Slit lamp examination—confirmatory
    - *Examples*: Refractive error, cataract, keratitis, uveitis, vitreous hemorrhage, glaucoma, etc.
- *Macula*:
    - Pinhole test—negative
    - Red reflex—normal
    - Color vision—impaired
    - Metamorphopsias—present
    - RAPD may be present.
    - *Examples*: Macular hole, macular degeneration, central serous retinopathy, and retinal dystrophies.
- *Retina*:
    - *Same as macula*: However, in severe retinal disease involving posterior lobe, the red reflex can be abnormal.
    - The retina looks abnormal in fundoscopic examination
    - *Examples*: Retinal detachment, retinal vascular occlusions, toxic retinopathies, carcinoma, and melanoma-associated paraneoplastic retinopathies.
- *Anterior visual pathway (i.e., optic nerve head to chiasma)*:
    - Monocular (sometimes binocular) vision loss/impairment
    - RAPD—present
    - Central scotoma and altitudinal field defect in one eye
    - Color vision—impaired.
    - *Fundoscopic examination*: In papillitis, disk margin is blurred and the disk is red in color. On the other hand, in optic atrophy, disk margin is well-defined and the disk is pale in color. If the fundus is normal and yet the patient complains of loss of vision, it must be a case of retrobulbar optic neuritis.

TABLE 30: Causes of optic nerve lesion.

Vascular	• Ischemic optic neuropathy • *Arteritic*: Giant-cell arteritis, SLE, PAN • *Non-arteritic*: Atherosclerosis
Demyelinating	• Multiple sclerosis • NMO spectrum disorder • MOG antibody disease
Inflammatory	*Optic neuritis*: • *Noninfectious*: ADEM • *Infectious*: Tuberculosis, HIV, syphilis, and Lyme disease
Neoplastic/nonneoplastic	• Pituitary tumor • Optic nerve sheath meningioma
Others	Toxic/nutritional/traumatic

(ADEM: acute disseminated encephalomyelitis; HIV: human immunodeficiency virus; MOG: myelin oligodendrocyte glycoprotein; NMO: neuromyelitis optica, PAN: polyarteritis nodosa; SLE: systemic lupus erythematosus)

- *Localization of optic nerve lesion:*
  - In orbit—isolated optic neuropathy
  - In optic canal or in intracranial portion—additional cranial nerves (IIIrd, IVth, and VIth) are involved.
  - Lesion close to optic chiasma—junctional scotoma is present.

The various causes of optic nerve lesion are enlisted in **Table 30**.[65]

Q27. What is the approach to a patient with acute onset bilateral loss of vision?

Ans. Acute onset bilateral loss of vision is either due to a bilateral optic nerve lesion or a lesion in the posterior visual pathway (i.e., chiasma or retrochiasmal lesion).

The following clinical features help us to localize the lesion in the posterior visual pathway:
- No RAPD
- Visual field examination—abrupt change across the vertical meridian in both eyes (homonymous/heteronymous hemianopias).
- Color vision—may be impaired
- Fundoscopic examination—usually normal

In bilateral loss of vision, look out for the following causes:
- Methyl alcohol poisoning
- Posterior reversible encephalopathy syndrome (PRES)
- Eclampsia
- Neuromyelitis optica (NMO)—spectrum disorder and myelin oligodendrocyte glycoprotein (MOG)—antibody disease
- Stroke[65]

Q28. Discuss the approach to a patient with facial pain.

Ans. Facial pain is one of the most frequent, yet one of the most confusing presenting symptoms for a physician. While eliciting history, try and know about the laterality, distribution of pain, whether it is paroxysmal/constant, its precipitating and relieving factors, trigger points, associated neurological signs and previous h/o neuroablative procedures. A strict unilaterality should arouse suspicion of psychogenic cause, whereas, spread to other side is indicative of a local pathology, e.g., maxillary sinusitis. With the exception of thalamic pain and atypical pain syndromes, neurologically relevant conditions usually cause pain restricted between vertex and lower border of mandible. Common conditions responsible for facial pain and some of their salient identifying features have been enlisted here:

- *Trigeminal neuralgia*: Unilateral, electric shock-like or lancinating pain limited to the distribution of one or more trigeminal nerves. The pain may be evoked by eating, drinking, talking, or even touching an area of the face, or may be spontaneous.
- *Glossopharyngeal neuralgia*: Unilateral, throat pain precipitated by drinking. It may be accompanied by additional pain in base of tongue, tonsillar fossa, angle of mandible, and ear as well as syncope or swallow syncope.
- *Postherpetic neuralgia*: Burning, itching, or stabbing unilateral pain typically within 90 days of herpes infection.
- Nervus intermedius: Unilateral, sharp episodic pain deep in the external ear
- *Ramsay Hunt syndrome*: VIIth and VIIIth nerve palsies with painful vesicular eruptions in the external ear.
- Short-lasting, unilateral, neuralgiform headache with conjunctival injection and tearing (SUNCT) and cluster headache—scope of detailed discussion is limited. But usually, they are most commonly identified by accompanying autonomic features.
- *Atypical facial pain*: Although described variably as a medically unexplained symptom, a "dustbin" diagnosis of exclusion, a manifestation of somatoform disorder, and atypical facial pain in itself is a distinct disease entity. It is characterized by no objective signs, inconclusive investigation reports, no identifiable cause, and a poor response to attempted treatments.
- *Others*: Giant-cell arteritis, cranial nerve disorders (optic neuritis, oculomotor palsies, temporomandibular pain disorders, and nasopharyngeal carcinoma)—look for masticatory muscle wasting, signs of other cranial nerve palsies, serous otitis media, cervical lymphadenopathy, proptosis, lid edema, and bruits. Never forget to exclude nasopharyngeal carcinoma as an etiology of facial pain.
- Ocular pain (acute glaucoma and eye strain headache)
- *Anesthesia dolorosa*: A very severe and difficult to treat condition following destructive procedures for trigeminal neuralgia, e.g., surgical rhizotomy, radiosurgery, etc.[80,81]

Q29. What is the approach to a patient with deviation of angle of mouth?

Ans. Deviation of angle of mouth is most commonly because of a facial nerve palsy on the opposite side. Less often, it can be due to a hemifacial spasm on account of irritation of the facial nerve of the same side in its intra-axial or extra-axial course.

It is important to differentiate whether the facial nerve palsy is an upper motor neuron (UMN) or lower motor neuron (LMN) lesion.

In an UMN lesion, voluntary movements of lower portion of face contralateral to the site of lesion are paralyzed. Upper part of face (frontalis and orbicularis oculi) is spared. This is because the motor neurons innervating the upper part of face receive bilateral projections from the cerebral hemispheres, while those supplying the lower part of face receive contralateral projections.

In an LMN lesion, the entire half of the face on the same side of lesion is paralyzed. Depending on clinical clues, the site of lesion can be further zeroed in as follows:

A. *Brainstem*:
- *Facial nucleus and fascicle*: Ipsilateral LMN VIIth nerve weakness plus horizontal gaze palsy [due to VIth nuclear or paramedian pontine reticular formation (PPRF) involvement] and contralateral hemiparesis.
- *Eight-and-a-half syndrome*: A lesion in dorsal tegmentum of caudal pons involving PPRF or VIth nerve nucleus, medial longitudinal fasciculus (MLF), and VIIth nerve nucleus or fascicle results in ipsilateral internuclear ophthalmoplegia (INO) plus ipsilateral horizontal gaze palsy (one-and-a-half syndrome) plus ipsilateral peripheral VIIth nerve palsy.
- In brainstem, there is anatomical separation of the motor fibers from the sensory and parasympathetic components. This explains why brainstem lesions may produce facial paralysis with sparing of taste and tearing.

B. *Cisternal segment (subarachnoid space)*:
- Isolated LMN VIIth palsy or combined with other cranial nerve involvement
- Meningeal signs may be present.
- Cerebellopontine (CP) angle lesions are associated with ipsilateral VIIth (including loss of taste in anterior two-thirds of tongue) and VIIIth nerve involvement (tinnitus, vertigo, and deafness) plus ipsilateral ataxia (cerebellar peduncle/cerebellar involvement) plus ipsilateral sensory symptoms/sign in face (due to Vth nerve involvement)
- *Examples*:
  - Infiltration of subarachnoid space by infection/neoplastic lesions
  - Guillain-Barré (GB) syndrome/Miller Fisher syndrome
  - CP angle lesion (e.g., meningioma, acoustic schwannoma, etc.)

C. *Intratemporal segment*:
   i. *Lesion at or just above the stylomastoid foramen*—weakness of muscles of facial expression on the same side.
   ii. *Lesion above the origin of chorda tympani*—all signs and symptoms of lesion (i) plus diminished taste sensation and salivation in anterior two-thirds of tongue
   iii. *Lesion above the origin of nerve to stapedius*—same as lesion (ii) plus hyperacusis
   iv. *Lesion at geniculate ganglion*—same as lesion (iii) plus loss of lacrimation
   v. *Lesion at meatal part*—facial nerve palsy is accompanied by hearing loss due to its close proximity to VIIIth cranial nerve.
   vi. *Examples*:
      - Bell's palsy—though Bell's palsy is the most common cause of LMN VIIth nerve palsy, every case of LMN facial palsy is not due to Bell's palsy.
      - *Ramsay Hunt syndrome*: Due to varicella zoster virus infection of geniculate ganglion—presents with LMN VIIth nerve palsy [as in site (iv) lesion] plus vesicular otic or oral rash with or without vestibulocochlear symptoms.
      - Gradenigo's syndrome—inflammation of petrous apex (facial nerve palsy plus Vth and VIth nerve palsy)
      - Traumatic fractures of temporal bone, occult skull-based neoplasms of temporal bone, complicated otitis media, and intratemporal facial nerve schwannoma within facial canal.

D. *Peripheral segment (facial nerve branch)*:
   - Lesion of facial nerve branch may cause weakness of selective facial muscles (may mimic UMN VIIth nerve weakness)
   - Taste, hearing, and lacrimation not affected
   - *Examples*: Parotid neoplasm, surgical procedures in face, and infiltrative skin cancers along VIIth nerve branch.[65]

Q30. What is the approach to a patient with deafness?

Ans. Deafness or hearing loss falls into two broad categories: (1) conductive [conductive hearing loss (CHL)] and (2) sensorineural [sensorineural hearing loss (SNHL)]. A defective conduction of sound to the cochlea, for example, disorder of external or middle ear or abnormality of the ossicular chain (e.g., otosclerosis) is responsible for conductive deafness. Sensorineural deafness is a result of disorders of the cochlea, cochlear nerve, or the central auditory pathways.

History can hint toward one of these categories, but to confirm the diagnosis, tuning fork tests need to be performed **(Table 31)**.

Conductive hearing loss can have various etiologies:

- Disorders of external ear, e.g., wax, foreign body, and otitis externa
- Disorders of middle ear, e.g., otitis media and mass in middle ear

TABLE 31: Differences between conductive and sensorineural deafness.

	Conductive deafness	Sensorineural deafness
History	Patients hear better in a noisy background than in a quiet setting	Patient complains of greater difficulty in hearing high-pitched sounds and vowels (e and i to a greater extent than a, o, or u)
Rinne's test: (Normal: AC is better than BC—Rinne test is positive)	AC is impaired but BC is normal (Rinne test is negative)	Both AC and BC are equally decreased but AC remains greater than BC (reduced Rinne positive)
Weber's test: (Normal: Bone conducted vibration is perceived equally in both ears (no lateralization).	Vibration is perceived louder in the deaf ear as inference from ambient sounds is muted on the affected side (lateralization to the deaf ear).	Vibrations are perceived louder in the normal ear (lateralization to the normal ear).
Schwabach's test: (Normal: Patient and examiner appreciate no difference)	BC normal or prolonged (the patient may hear the tuning fork longer than the examiner does).	BC worse in patient than the examiner

(AC: air conduction; BC: bone conduction)

If CHL is suspected, the patient is to be referred to an ENT specialist for further evaluation.

Sensorineural hearing loss can be further localized on the basis of clues from **Table 32**.[65]

Q31. How to choose preventive drugs for migraine?

Ans. Preventive medications for migraine are considered in chronic migraines (15 or more days of headaches per month), frequent migraines (>4–5 attacks per month), migraines are infrequent but highly debilitating, difficulty tolerating or having a contraindication to acute therapy, medication-overuse headache or the presence of certain migraine subtypes (i.e., hemiplegic migraine; migraine with brainstem aura; migrainous infarction; or frequent, persistent, or uncomfortable aura symptoms).[82,83] The goal is to reduce the frequency, duration, and severity of attacks.

Migraine therapy is started with medications that have the highest level of evidence-based effectiveness. Medications are chosen based on headache frequency, anticipated side effects and comorbidities, and living conditions (e.g., shift work) and response to previous treatments. Agents are avoided that are contraindicated or that may exacerbate coexisting conditions. Medications are started with the lowest effective dose and titrate every 2–4 weeks until therapeutic effect or until patient develops adverse effects. Successful treatment is defined as a 50% reduction in the number of headache attacks or days, a significant decrease in the duration of attacks, or an improvement in response to acute therapy. if no response occurs after

TABLE 32: Localization of SNHL.

Localization	Clinical clues	Etiologies
Cochlea	Abnormally heightened perception of loudness with an increase in the intensity of the stimulus, i.e., loudness recruitment	• Meniere's disease • Advanced otosclerosis • Prolonged exposure to loud noise • Ototoxic drugs • Internal auditory artery occlusions
Cochlear division of VIIIth nerve	• Uniform decrease in hearing of both high and low intensity sounds • Poor speech discrimination	• Acoustic neuroma • Meningioma • Epidermoid • Vascular loops • Transverse temporal bone fracture • Meningitis
Cerebellopontine angle	• Ipsilateral Vth, VIth, VIIth, IXth, and Xth cranial nerves involved • Ipsilateral cerebellar signs • Contralateral hemiplegia • Bruns nystagmus	• Acoustic neuroma • Meningioma • Epidermoid • Meningitis
Brainstem	Deafness due to brainstem lesion is rare as a lesion needs to be massive to interrupt both the crossed and uncrossed projections from the cochlear nuclei	
Cerebrum	As cochlear nucleus is connected with cortex of both temporal lobes, a unilateral or even bilateral cerebral lesion usually does not cause deafness. However, the patient may develop pure word deafness (auditory verbal agnosia) characterized by inability to understand the spoken language in spite of normal auditory acuity.	Stroke Demyelination Tumor

2 months, therapy should be changed.[82] For calcitonin gene-related peptide (CGRP) inhibitors, efficacy should be assessed only after 3–6 months while for onabotulinum toxin A, efficacy should be assessed after 6–9 months.[84]

Topiramate, valproic acid, propranolol, bisoprolol, metoprolol, flunarizine, amitriptyline, CGRP inhibitors, candesartan, and onabotulinum toxin A (approved only in chronic migraine) are medications for migraine prevention with high/good scientific evidence while acetylsalicylic acid (ASA), magnesium, coenzyme Q10, and angiotensin-converting enzyme (ACE) inhibitors (lisinopril) have less scientific evidence.[84,85]

Table 33 is a summary of the classes of preventive drugs for migraines with their advantages, side effects, and contraindications:[83,85,86]

TABLE 33: Drugs classes of preventive drugs for migraines with their advantages, side effects, and contraindications.

Drug class	Examples	Advantages	Side effects	Contraindications
CGRP Inhibitors	Erenumab, eptinezumab, fremanezumab, galcanezumab (CGRP mAbs) Atogepant Rimegepant (gepants)	New class proven to reduce migraine frequency and severity. First-line option for migraine prevention Effective for both episodic and chronic migraine Can be effective after failure of conventional therapies	Injection site reactions (pain and redness), constipation, fatigue, and mild allergic reactions Nasopharyngitis, angioedema, urticaria, and facial flushing (eptinezumab)	Hypersensitivity to the drug, pregnancy (safety not well established)
Antiseizure medications	Topiramate	Beneficial for obesity (weight loss effect) and patients with epilepsy	Fatigue, cognitive impairment, weight loss, paresthesias, impaired taste, psychosis, kidney stones, depression, and narrow-angle glaucoma	Absolute: Renal insufficiency, kidney stones, and narrow-angle glaucoma. Relative: Depression, anxiety disorder, low body weight, and anorexia
	Valproate	Useful when migraine occurs in those with epilepsy, anxiety disorders, or bipolar disease	Fatigue, dizziness, tremor, skin rash, alopecia, weight gain, and impaired liver function	Impaired liver function, pregnancy (neural tube defects), women of childbearing potential, and alcohol abuse
β-blockers	Propranolol, metoprolol, and bisoprolol	Beneficial for patients with hypertension, heart disease, and anxiety attack	Fatigue, dizziness, lightheadedness, bradycardia, bronchospasm, hypotension, depression, sleep disturbances, and erectile dysfunction	Asthma, COPD (worsens bronchoconstriction), bradycardia, heart block, and severe depression

Continued

Continued

Drug class	Examples	Advantages	Side effects	Contraindications
Antidepressants	Amitriptyline, Venlafaxine, Nortriptyline	Effective for migraines with coexisting depression or anxiety Can help with sleep problems that may trigger migraines	Sedation, dry mouth, constipation, weight gain, orthostatic hypotension, dizziness, blurred vision, and sexual dysfunction	Glaucoma, urinary retention, heart disease (for tricyclics such as amitriptyline), and recent heart attack (especially venlafaxine)
Calcium channel blockers	Flunarizine	Useful in prolonged or complicated migraine aura Effective for migraine prevention in children	Fatigue, weight gain, gastrointestinal complaints, depression, hyperkinesias, tremor, and parkinsonoid	Focal dystonia, pregnancy, lactation, depression, and Parkinson in the family
Botulinum toxin	Onabotulinum toxin A	Effective for chronic migraines Nonsystemic (injected around the head and neck)	Injection site pain, bruising, neck pain, muscle weakness, difficulty swallowing, and drooping eyelids (rare)	Pregnancy, breastfeeding, neurological disorders (e.g., myasthenia gravis), allergic reactions to botulinum toxin, and anticoagulation
Angiotensin-receptor blockers	Candesartan	Useful in patients with arterial hypertension	Dizziness, headache, and angioneurotic edema	Impaired kidney function, valvular defect, cardiomyopathy, pregnancy, and lactation
Supplements	Magnesium, riboflavin, coenzyme Q10 (CoQ10)	Nonprescription, can be used as adjunctive therapy.	Magnesium: Diarrhea (if excessive). Riboflavin: Yellow-orange urine. CoQ10: Mild gastrointestinal upset.	Magnesium: Caution with kidney disease. Riboflavin and CoQ10: Generally safe but avoid if allergic to B2.

(COPD: chronic obstructive pulmonary disease; mAbs: monoclonal antibodies)

Preventive Medicines in Special Considerations

Prevention of Migraine Aura

Lamotrigine is not effective in the reduction of migraine attack frequency, but it may reduce the frequency of migraine attacks with aura. Flunarizine is effective in a reduction in frequency of both auras and migraine attacks. In some cases, topiramate is also effective. An effect of acetazolamide or lamotrigine, also in combination with valproic acid, has been described for sporadic or familiar hemiplegic migraine.[85]

Menstrual-associated Migraine

Around 8% of women experience migraines exclusively related to menstruation, known as pure menstrual migraine. Daily use of a long-acting nonsteroidal anti-inflammatory drug (NSAID) (e.g., naproxen) or triptan (e.g., frovatriptan, naratriptan, and zolmitriptan) for 5 days, starting 2 days before menstruation, can effectively prevent migraines. Continuous use of combined hormonal contraceptives may help prevent pure menstrual migraine without aura but is contraindicated in women with migraine with aura due to an increased stroke risk.[84]

Children

Only flunarizine has sufficient evidence to be considered probably effective for migraine prevention in children. Medications such as propranolol and topiramate have conflicting results in studies. Agents, including cyproheptadine, amitriptyline, valproic acid, and levetiracetam, have insufficient data in children.[83]

Pregnancy and breastfeeding women

Nonpharmacologic options are preferred before drug therapy in pregnancy. β-blockers, such as propranolol and amitriptyline if propranolol is contraindicated, are generally safe.[84] Valproic acid should be avoided due to teratogenic risks, as should topiramate and ACE inhibitors due to potential fetal harm. Migraine treatments during the postpartum period should be used cautiously to protect the infant. If preventive medication is necessary, propranolol is the first choice due to its favorable safety profile.[84,87]

Q32. First seizure episode with no underlying causes, normal electroencephalogram (EEG), and MRI—How to proceed?

Once an acute provoking cause has been excluded, the next step is to decide if the first seizure indicated a focal or generalized epilepsy syndrome, what is the recurrence risk and what sort of activity restrictions are needed—a critical distinction if drug treatment is considered.[88] The most consistent factors associated with an increased risk of seizure recurrence following an unprovoked first seizure include a prior brain lesion or insult, EEG with epileptiform abnormalities, significant brain-imaging abnormality, and a nocturnal seizure. In children, the presence of Todd's paresis, global developmental delay, or intellectual disability augmented the possibility of recurrence.[89,90]

In patients with history of prior brain insult should be asked for imaging preferably magnetic resonance imaging (MRI). According to a study, EEG should be executed within the first 16 hours after seizure onset. When standard EEG is negative, systematic case series have shown that sleep deprived EEG will detect epileptiform (spike) discharges in an additional 13–31% of cases.[88]

As there is no general rule, the decision to start antiseizure medication (ASM) treatment following a first unprovoked seizure should be individualized and based on patient preference, clinical, chance of recurrence, legal, and sociocultural factors.

Antiseizure medication may be justified when the risk of recurrence is high, such as with a focal structural brain deficit and corresponding EEG epileptiform activity, epilepsy syndrome, when the risk of injury from a recurrent seizure is high (such as for those with a spinal cervical fracture, with severe osteoporosis, or taking anticoagulants); or when the risk of economic hardship from a recurrence is high (such as loss of employment). If drug treatment is started after a first seizure, at least 6 months to 1 year of treatment is required.[88]

When both MRI and EEG are normal, epilepsy syndrome is unlikely and no other risk factor is present, decision to start ASM depends upon patient preference and socioeconomical factor. Patient should be educated that chance for a recurrent seizure is greatest within the first 2 years after a first seizure (21–45%), antiepileptic drug (AED) may reduce the risk for a seizure recurrence but may not improve quality of life (QOL). Patients should be told that their risk for ASM adverse effects ranges from 7 to 31% and that these adverse effects are predominantly mild and reversible.[91]

Typically, starting an ASM is not warranted in this situation. Patients should be followed and monitored regularly for new symptoms or any event. Patients and family members should be taught triggering factors and safety tips. Midazolam spray can be prescribed. Restrictions to recreational activity after a first untreated, unprovoked seizure should be individualized and limited to 2 or 3 months for children and adults. Swimming, scuba diving, and climbing may carry a higher risk of injury than do cross-country skiing, long-distance running, or soccer. Patients should probably be suspended from working with dangerous machines for at least 6 months. Laws regarding the suspension of a driving license after a first seizure vary between countries from no restriction to 1 year.[88,90]

Q33. When to refer a patient with PD for intervention?

Indications for referral for DBS: See Table 34.

Indications for Referral for Lesioning Procedures:[93]

- *Targeted symptom management*:
    - Focal symptoms such as severe tremor that do not respond to medications.
    - Patients with tremor-dominant PD who are not DBS candidates.

TABLE 34: Refer for DBS—indications and prerequisites.[92]

Category	Details
Indications:	
Motor complications	• Persistent motor fluctuations and dyskinesias despite optimal medical therapy • "5-2-1" criteria (as screening): ○ 5: Taking five doses of levodopa daily ○ 2: Experiencing ≥2 hours of "off" time daily ○ 1: Having ≥1 hour of troublesome dyskinesia daily
Tremor refractory to treatment	Levodopa-resistant tremor unresponsive to a daily LEDD ≥ 900 mg.
Intolerance to dopaminergic agents	Adverse effects preventing dose escalation (e.g., somnolence, hypotension, impulse control disorders, and psychosis)
Prerequisites:	
Confirmed diagnosis	PD diagnosis consistent with Movement Disorder Society criteria. Atypical parkinsonism is excluded.
Minimum disease duration	≥4 years since disease onset to avoid operating on atypical parkinsonism
Levodopa response	≥33% improvement in symptoms during a levodopa challenge
Cognitive and psychiatric health	No severe cognitive impairment or uncontrolled neuropsychiatric conditions
Postoperative commitment	Regular follow-up attendance and reliable social support for rehabilitation and device adjustments

(DBS: deep brain stimulation; LEDD: levodopa equivalent daily dose; PD: Parkinson's disease)

- *Unavailability of DBS*:
  - DBS contraindicated due to advanced age, cognitive decline, or high surgical risks.
  - Limited access to DBS resources or patient preference against an implantable device

Q34. What is the approach to rapidly progressive dementia?

Rapidly progressive dementia (RPD) refers to a cognitive decline that progresses significantly faster than typical dementias, often leading to near-complete dependency within weeks to months and rarely exceeding 1–2 years. Although rare, RPD requires an urgent and systematic approach to identify treatable causes and optimize patient outcomes **(Table 35)**. Common causes span a broad spectrum, for which Mnemonic tools (e.g., VITAMINS) may be useful.[94]

A detailed clinical history from both the patient and reliable informants is essential to identify risk factors, progression patterns, and relevant exposures. This is complemented by a comprehensive neurological and systemic examination to localize the pathology and determine whether the process is focal, multifocal, or systemic **(Tables 36 and 37)**.

A stepwise diagnostic approach is key, starting with screening tests such as basic laboratory panels, neuroimaging (MRI preferred), cerebrospinal fluid (CSF) analysis, and EEG. These tests aim to exclude common conditions and identify red flags such as inflammation, structural abnormalities, or biomarkers of specific diseases. Targeted tests, including antibody panels for autoimmune encephalitis, advanced imaging [e.g., fluorodeoxyglucose-positron emission tomography (FDG-PET) for malignancies], and genetic studies, are guided by clinical suspicion. In select cases where noninvasive diagnostics fail, tissue biopsies may be necessary **(Table 38)**.

Timely recognition of reversible causes is crucial. For example, autoimmune encephalitis may present with prominent psychiatric or seizure symptoms, which are often mistaken for primary psychiatric illnesses. Prompt initiation of empiric therapy, such as steroids or antivirals, is warranted when treatable conditions such as infections/inflammation are suspected.

TABLE 35: Common causes of RPD.[94,95]

Category	Examples
Vascular	Infarcts and vasculitis
Infectious	Creutzfeldt–Jakob disease, neurosyphilis, HIV encephalopathy, SSPE, and meningitis/encephalitis
Toxins/metabolic	Heavy metals, recreational drug use, Wernicke–Korsakoff syndrome, and hepatic encephalopathy
Autoimmune/ inflammatory	NMDA receptor encephalitis, LGI1 antibody encephalitis, granulomatous disease (e.g., sarcoidosis), and cerebral amyloid angiopathy with related inflammation
Malignancy	CNS lymphoma, primary CNS tumor, metastasis, and paraneoplastic syndromes
Iatrogenic	Medications (anticholinergics, benzodiazepines, and neuroleptics), extrapontine myelinolysis, and radiation-induced leukoencephalopathy
Neurodegenerative	Alzheimer's, Lewy body dementia, frontotemporal dementia
Systemic/structural	Hypoxia/hypercarbia and hydrocephalus (normal or high pressure)

(CNS: central nervous system; HIV: human immunodeficiency virus; LGI1: leucine-rich glioma inactivated 1; NMDA: N-methyl-D-aspartate; RPD: rapidly progressive dementia; SSPE: subacute sclerosing panencephalitis)

TABLE 36: Clinical clues in history for rapidly progressive dementia (RPD).[94,95]

Category	Clinical clues
Onset and progression	Abrupt onset (vascular and infectious); subacute onset over weeks (autoimmune and inflammatory); steady decline (CJD)
Age of onset	Young age (autoimmune, inherited leukoencephalopathies, inborn errors of metabolism); older age (neurodegenerative, vascular, and sporadic CJD)
Sex	Female: Autoimmune diseases (e.g., lupus) Male: LGI1 encephalitis and CJD
Medical history	Autoimmune diseases, cancer (paraneoplastic syndromes), and vascular risk factors (hypertension and diabetes)
Infectious risk factors	Travel to endemic areas, insect/animal bites, high-risk sexual behavior (HIV and neurosyphilis), and immunosuppression
Family history	Early-onset dementia, autosomal dominant inheritance (e.g., PRNP mutation and frontotemporal dementia)
Drug and toxin exposure	Immunosuppressants (opportunistic infections), heavy metals, and recreational drugs
Psychiatric symptoms	Early psychosis (NMDA receptor encephalitis); mood swings or disinhibition (frontotemporal dementia)

(CJD: Creutzfeldt–Jakob disease; HIV: human immunodeficiency virus; LGI1: leucine-rich glioma inactivated 1; NMDA: N-methyl-D-aspartate)

TABLE 37: Clinical clues in examination for rapidly progressive dementia (RPD).[94,95]

Category	Clinical clues
General physical examination	Cachexia (malignancy and nutritional deficiency); fever/meningismus (infection); skin/joint changes (autoimmune diseases)
Cognitive and psychiatric	Prominent psychosis (autoimmune encephalitis); apathy or disinhibition (frontotemporal dementia)
Motor signs	Myoclonus (CJD and metabolic encephalopathy); faciobrachial dystonic seizures (LGI1 encephalitis); rigidity (parkinsonism)
Focal neurologic deficits	Hemiparesis, visual loss, and sensory deficits (vascular or neoplastic causes)
Cranial nerve examination	Ophthalmoplegia (Wernicke's and brainstem lesion); Horner syndrome (Pancoast tumor)
Systemic signs	Lymphadenopathy, organomegaly (paraneoplastic); stigmata of liver disease (hepatic encephalopathy)

(CJD: Creutzfeldt–Jakob disease; LGI1: leucine-rich glioma inactivated 1)

TABLE 38: Testing Approach for RPD.[94,95]

Test type	Purpose	Examples/details
Screening tests	Identify metabolic, infectious, or toxic causes	Serum: CBC, electrolytes, liver/kidney function, thyroid panel, vitamin B12, folate, HIV, and syphilis tests
Neuroimaging	Detect structural lesions, inflammation, or ischemic changes	MRI (preferred) with DWI, T2/FLAIR; consider CT for emergencies
CSF analysis	Evaluate infections, inflammation, or prion disease	Cell count, glucose, protein, oligoclonal bands, prion biomarkers (RT-QuIC), and tau levels
EEG	Identify seizures or encephalopathy	Look for slowing, periodic complexes (e.g., Creutzfeldt–Jakob disease), or seizure activity
Autoimmune testing	Diagnose autoimmune encephalitis	CSF and serum antibodies: NMDA receptor, LGI1, CASPR2, Hu, Ma, and GAD65
Infectious workup	Detect specific pathogens	PCR or serology for herpes simplex, JC virus, TB; cultures as indicated
Biomarker testing	Support neurodegenerative or prion diseases	CSF: tau, Aβ42/Aβ40 ratios, and neurofilament light chain
Genetic testing	Evaluate inherited conditions	PRNP mutations for prion disease; C9orf72 for frontotemporal dementia
Advanced imaging	Explore systemic causes	FDG-PET for malignancies; CT or ultrasound for paraneoplastic syndrome
Biopsy	Confirm diagnosis when other methods fail	Brain biopsy for suspected lymphoma or vasculitis; skin/muscle biopsy for systemic diseases

(CBC: complete blood count; CSF: cerebrospinal fluid; CT: computed tomography; DWI: diffusion-weighted imaging; EEG: electroencephalogram; FDG-PET: fluorodeoxyglucose-positron emission tomography; FLAIR: fluid-attenuated inversion recovery; HIV: human immunodeficiency virus; JC: John Cunningham; LGI1: leucine-rich glioma inactivated 1; MRI: magnetic resonance imaging; NMDA: N-methyl-D-aspartate; PCR: PCR: polymerase chain reaction; RPD: rapidly progressive dementia; TB: tuberculosis)

REFERENCES

1. Yiannopoulou KG, Papageorgiou SG. Current and future treatments in Alzheimer disease: an update. Journal of central nervous system disease. 2020;12:1179573520907397.
2. Schmidt R, Hofer E, Bouwman FH, Buerger K, Cordonnier C, Fladby T, et al. EFNS-ENS/EAN Guideline on concomitant use of cholinesterase inhibitors and memantine in moderate to severe Alzheimer's disease. Eur J Neurol. 2015;22(6):889-98.
3. Jones RW. Drug treatment for people with dementia. Clinical medicine. 2011;11(1):67.
4. Correll CU, Martin A, Patel C, Benson C, Goulding R, Kern-Sliwa J, et al. Systematic literature review of schizophrenia clinical practice guidelines on acute and maintenance management with antipsychotics. Schizophrenia. 2022;8(1):5.

5. Gardner DM, Baldessarini RJ, Waraich P. Modern antipsychotic drugs: a critical overview. CMAJ. 2005;172(13):1703-11.
6. Joyce EM. Organic psychosis: the pathobiology and treatment of delusions. CNS Neurosci Ther. 2018;24(7):598-603.
7. Faden J. How do we select an antipsychotic for those with schizophrenia?. Expert Opin Pharmacother. 2019;20(18):2195-9.
8. Hiremath SB, Gautam AA, Sasindran V, Therakathu J, Benjamin G. Cerebrospinal fluid rhinorrhea and otorrhea: A multimodality imaging approach. Diagn Intervent Imaging. 2019;100(1):3-15.
9. Oakley GM, Alt JA, Schlosser RJ, Harvey RJ, Orlandi RR. Diagnosis of cerebrospinal fluid rhinorrhea: an evidence-based review with recommendations. Intern Forum Allergy Rhinol. 2016;6(1):8-16.
10. Mathias T, Levy J, Fatakia A, McCoul ED. Contemporary approach to the diagnosis and management of cerebrospinal fluid rhinorrhea. Ochsner J. 2016;16(2):136-42.
11. Prosser JD, Vender JR, Solares CA. Traumatic cerebrospinal fluid leaks. Otolaryngol Clin North Am. 2011;44(4):857-73.
12. Dalmau J, Armangué T, Planagumà J, Radosevic M, Mannara F, Leypoldt F, et al. An update on anti-NMDA receptor encephalitis for neurologists and psychiatrists: mechanisms and models. Lancet Neurol. 2019;18(11):1045-57.
13. Lyketsos CG, Kozauer N, Rabins PV. Psychiatric manifestations of neurologic disease: where are we headed?. Dialog Clin Neurosci. 2007;9(2):111-24.
14. Welch KA, Carson AJ. When psychiatric symptoms reflect medical conditions. Clin Med. 2018;18(1):80-7.
15. Ng IK, Chua JW, Lui YS, Tan LF, Teo DB. Approach to acute psychosis in older adults. Singapore Med J. 2023;64(6):391-7.
16. Zun LS. Approach to the Psychiatric Patient. In: Sherman SC, Weber JM, Schindlbeck MA, Rahul GP (Eds). Clinical Emergency Medicine. New York, NY: McGraw-Hill Education; 2014.
17. Chia KY, Tey HL. Approach to hypohidrosis. Journal of the European Acad Dermatol Venereol. 2013;27(7):799-804.
18. Schlereth T, Dieterich M, Birklein F. Hyperhidrosis—causes and treatment of enhanced sweating. Dtsch Arztebl Int. 2009;106(3):32-7.
19. Cheshire WP. Sudomotor dysfunction. In: David MG, Albin CSW, Kimchi EY (Eds). Seminars in Neurology. Thieme Medical Publishers; 2020. pp. 560-8).
20. Kempler P, Amarenco G, Freeman R, Frontoni S, Horowitz M, Stevens M, et al. Management strategies for gastrointestinal, erectile, bladder, and sudomotor dysfunction in patients with diabetes. Diabetes/Metabol Res Rev. 2011;27(7):665-77.
21. Low PA. Testing the autonomic nervous system. In: David MG, Albin CSW, Kimchi EY (Eds). Seminars in Neurology. Thieme Medical Publishers; 2020. pp. 407-422.
22. Illigens BM, Gibbons CH. Sweat testing to evaluate autonomic function. Clinical Autonomic Research. 2009;19:79-87.
23. Quinton PM. Sweating and its disorders. Ann Rev Med. 1983;34(1):429-52.
24. Muncie HL, Sirmans SM, James E. Dizziness: approach to evaluation and management. American family physician. 2017;95(3):154-62.
25. Hain TC, Uddin M. Pharmacological treatment of vertigo. CNS Drugs. 2003;17:85-100.
26. Swartz R, Longwell P. Treatment of vertigo. Am Fam Phys. 2005;71(6):1115-22.
27. Viola P, Gioacchini FM, Astorina A, Pisani D, Scarpa A, Marcianò G, et al. The pharmacological treatment of acute vestibular syndrome. Front Neurol. 2022;13:999112.
28. Gold DR, Morris L, Kheradmand A, Schubert MC. Repositioning maneuvers for benign paroxysmal positional vertigo. Current treatment options in neurology. 2014;16:1-22.
29. Smyth D, Britton Z, Murdin L, Arshad Q, Kaski D. Vestibular migraine treatment: a comprehensive practical review. Brain. 2022;145(11):3741-54.
30. Sharif S, Khoujah D, Greer A, Naples JG, Upadhye S, Edlow JA. Vestibular suppressants for benign paroxysmal positional vertigo: A systematic review and meta-analysis of randomized controlled trials. Acad Emerg Med. 2023;30(5):541-51.

31. D'Antonio F, Boccia M, Di Vita A, Suppa A, Fabbrini A, Canevelli M, et al. Visual hallucinations in Lewy body disease: pathophysiological insights from phenomenology. J Neurol. 2022;269(7):3636-52.
32. O'Brien J, Taylor JP, Ballard C, Barker RA, Bradley C, Burns A, et al. Visual hallucinations in neurological and ophthalmological disease: pathophysiology and management. J Neurol Neurosurg Psychiatry. 2020;91(5):512-9.
33. Badcock JC, Larøi F, Kamp K, Kelsall-Foreman I, Bucks RS, Weinborn M, et al. Hallucinations in older adults: a practical review. Schizophr Bull. 2020;46(6):1382-95.
34. Weil RS, Lees AJ. Visual hallucinations. Pract Neurol. 2021;21(4):327-32.
35. Neubauer DN, Pandi-Perumal SR, Spence DW, Buttoo K, Monti JM. Pharmacotherapy of insomnia. J Cent Nerv Syst Dis. 2018;10:1179573518770672.
36. Chan NY, Chan JW, Li SX, Wing YK. Non-pharmacological approaches for management of insomnia. Neurotherapeutics. 2021;18(1):32-43.
37. Martin JL. Cognitive behavioral therapy for insomnia in adults., Waltham, MA: UpToDate; 2020. p. 12.
38. Holder S, Narula NS. Common sleep disorders in adults: Diagnosis and management. American family physician. 2022;105(4):397-405.
39. Krystal AD, Prather AA, Ashbrook LH. The assessment and management of insomnia: an update. World Psychiatry. 2019;18(3):337-52.
40. Bonsignore MR, Lombardi C, Lombardo S, Fanfulla F. Epidemiology, physiology and clinical approach to sleepiness at the wheel in OSA patients: a narrative review. J Clin Med. 2022;11(13):3691.
41. Roche F, Berger M. One excessive daytime sleepiness evaluation does not fit all: time to implement a multidimensional approach. Sleep. 2023;46(8):zsad021.
42. Gandhi KD, Mansukhani MP, Silber MH, Kolla BP. Excessive Daytime Sleepiness: A Clinical Review. Mayo Clin Proc. 2021;96(5):1288-1301.
43. Pérez-Carbonell L, Mignot E, Leschziner G, Dauvilliers Y. Understanding and approaching excessive daytime sleepiness. Lancet. 2022;400(10357):1033-46.
44. Pagel JF. Excessive daytime sleepiness. Am Fam Phys. 2009;79(5):391-6.
45. Brown J, Makker HK. An approach to excessive daytime sleepiness in adults. BMJ. 2020;368.
46. Murray BJ. A practical approach to excessive daytime sleepiness: a focused review. Can Respir J. 2016;2016(1):4215938.
47. Yaghi S, Willey JZ, Cucchiara B, Goldstein JN, Gonzales NR, Khatri P, et al. Treatment and outcome of hemorrhagic transformation after intravenous alteplase in acute ischemic stroke: a scientific statement for healthcare professionals from the American Heart Association/American Stroke Association. Stroke. 2017;48(12):e343-61.
48. Kim JT, Heo SH, Park MS, Chang J, Choi KH, Cho KH. Use of antithrombotics after hemorrhagic transformation in acute ischemic stroke. PLoS One. 2014;9(2):e89798.
49. Seiffge DJ, Werring DJ, Paciaroni M, Dawson J, Warach S, Milling TJ, et al. Timing of anticoagulation after recent ischaemic stroke in patients with atrial fibrillation. Lancet Neurol. 2019;18(1):117-26.
50. von Kummer R, Broderick JP, Campbell BC, Demchuk A, Goyal M, Hill MD, et al. The Heidelberg bleeding classification: classification of bleeding events after ischemic stroke and reperfusion therapy. Stroke. 2015;46(10):2981-6.
51. Makris M, Veen JJ, Tait CR, Mumford AD, Laffan M. Guideline on the management of bleeding in patients on antithrombotic agents. Br J Haematol. 2013;160(1).
52. El-Tallawy SN, Nalamasu R, Salem GI, LeQuang JA, Pergolizzi JV, Christo PJ. Management of musculoskeletal pain: an update with emphasis on chronic musculoskeletal pain. Pain Therapy. 2021;10:181-209.
53. Dolati S, Tarighat F, Pashazadeh F, Shahsavarinia K, Gholipouri S, Soleimanpour H. The role of opioids in pain management in elderly patients with chronic kidney disease: a review article. Anesthesiol Pain Med. 2020;10(5).
54. Pham PC, Khaing K, Sievers TM, Pham PM, Miller JM, Pham SV, et al. 2017 update on pain management in patients with chronic kidney disease. Clin Kidney J. 2017;10(5):688-97.

55. Lambourg E, Colvin L, Guthrie G, Murugan K, Lim M, Walker H, et al. The prevalence of pain among patients with chronic kidney disease using systematic review and meta-analysis. Kidney Intern. 2021;100(3):636-49.
56. Mirishova S, Hammad YM. Pain Management in Patients with Impaired Kidney Function. In: Shallik NA (Ed). Pain Management in Special Circumstances. IntechOpen; 2018.
57. Roy PJ, Weltman M, Dember LM, Liebschutz J, Jhamb M, HOPE Consortium. Pain management in patients with chronic kidney disease and end-stage kidney disease. Curr Opin Nephrol Hypertens. 2020;29(6):671-80.
58. Costa F, Oertel J, Zileli M, Restelli F, Zygourakis CC, Sharif S. Role of surgery in primary lumbar disk herniation: WFNS spine committee recommendations. World Neurosurg X. 2024;22:100276.
59. Sabnis AB, Diwan AD. The timing of surgery in lumbar disc prolapse: A systematic review. Indian J Orthop. 2014;48(2):127-35.
60. Yoon WW, Koch J. Herniated discs: when is surgery necessary? EFORT Open Rev. 2021;6(6):526-30.
61. Mula M, Kanner AM, Jetté N, Sander JW. Psychiatric Comorbidities in People with Epilepsy. Neurol Clin Pract. 2021;11(2):e112-e120.
62. Revdal E, Kolstad BP, Winsvold BS, Selmer KK, Morken G, Brodtkorb E. Psychiatric comorbidity in relation to clinical characteristics of epilepsy: A retrospective observational study. Seizure. 2023;110:136-43.
63. Kedare JS, Baliga SP. Management of Psychiatric Disorders in Patients of Epilepsy. Indian J Psychiatry. 2022;64(Suppl 2):S319-29.
64. Alrayes MS, Altawili M, Alsaffar MH, Alfarhan GZ, Owedah RJ, Bodal IS, et al. Surgical Interventions for the Management of Carpal Tunnel Syndrome: A Narrative Review. Cureus. 2024;16(3):e55593.
65. Ray BK. Bedside Neurology. New Delhi: Jaypee Brothers Medical Publishers; 2022.
66. Laska AC, Hellblom A, Murray V, Kahan T, Von Arbin M. Aphsia in acute stroke and relation to outcome. J Intern Med. 2001;249:413-22.
67. Pedersen PM, Jorgensen HS, Nakayama H, Raaschou HO, Olsen TS. Aphasia in acute stroke: incidence, determinants, and recovery. Ann Neurol. 1995;38:659-66.
68. Black-Schaffer RM, Osberg JS. Return towork after stroke: development of a predictive model. Arch Phys Med Rehabil. 1990;71:285-90.
69. Pohjasvaara T, Erkinjuntti T, Ylikoski R, Hietanen M, Vataja R, Kaste M. Clinical determinants of post-stroke dementia. Stroke 1998;29:75-81.
70. Wein T, Lindsay MP, Côté R, Foley N, Berlingieri J, et al. Canadian stroke best practice recommendations: secondary prevention of stroke, practice guidelines, update 2017. Int J Stroke. 2018;13(4):420-3.
71. Kim AS. Medical Management for Secondary Stroke Prevention. Continuum: Lifelong Learning in Neurology. 2020;26(2):435-56.
72. Practical Neurology. (2020). Diagnosing Secondary Headaches. [online] Available from https://practicalneurology.com/articles/2020-may/diagnosing-secondary-headaches/pdf [Last accessed January, 2025].
73. Whitehead S, Baalbergen E. Post-stroke rehabilitation. S Afr Med J. 2019;109(2):81-3.
74. O'Dell MW. Stroke rehabilitation and motor recovery. Continuum: Lifelong Learning in Neurology. 2023;29(2):605-27.
75. Wang CM, Wu BR, Xiang P, Xiao J, Hu XC. Management of male erectile dysfunction: From the past to the future. Front Endocrinol. 2023;14:1148834.
76. Dalrymple SN, Lewis SH, Philman S. Tinnitus: diagnosis and management. Am Fam Physician. 2021;103(11):663-71.
77. Ropper AH, Samuels MA, Klein J. Adams and Victor's Principles of Neurology, 11th edition. New York: McGraw-Hill Education; 2019.
78. Ranganathan LN. Localization of Clinical Neurology. Gurgaon, India: Wolters Kluwer India Pvt. Ltd.; 2020.

79. Beauchet O, Dubost V, Revel-Delhom C, Berrut G, Belmin J. How to manage recurrent falls in clinical practice: guidelines of the French Society of Geriatrics and Gerontology. J Nutr Health Aging. 2011;15:79-84.
80. Daroff RB, Jankovic J, Mazziotta JC, Pomeroy SL. Bradley's Neurology in Clinical Practice. London, New York, Oxford, Philadelphia, St Louis, Sydney, Toronto: Elsevier; 2016.
81. Chakravarty A. Case Studies in Uncommon Headache Disorders. New Delhi: Jaypee Brothers Medical Publishers; 2019.
82. Silberstein SD. Preventive migraine treatment. Continuum (Minneap Minn). 2015; 21(4 Headache):973-89.
83. Ha H, Gonzalez A. Migraine Headache Prophylaxis. Am Fam Physician. 2019;99(1):17-24.
84. Eigenbrodt AK, Ashina H, Khan S, Diener HC, Mitsikostas DD, Sinclair AJ, et al. Diagnosis and management of migraine in ten steps. Nat Rev Neurol. 2017;17:501-14.
85. Charles AC, Digre KB, Goadsby PJ, Robbins MS, Hershey A; American Headache Society. Calcitonin gene-related peptide-targeting therapies are a first-line option for the prevention of migraine: An American Headache Society position statement update. Headache. 2024;64(4):333-41.
86. Diener HC, Holle-Lee D, Nägel S, Dresler T, Gaul C, Göbel H, et al. et al. Treatment of migraine attacks and prevention of migraine: Guidelines by the German Migraine and Headache Society and the German Society of Neurology. Clin Transl Neurosci. 2019:1-40.
87. Amundsen S, Nordeng H, Nezvalová-Henriksen K, Stovner LJ, Spigset O. Pharmacological treatment of migraine during pregnancy and breastfeeding. Nat Rev Neurol. 2015;11: 209-19.
88. Pohlmann-Eden B, Beghi E, Camfield C, Camfield P. The first seizure and its management in adults and children. BMJ. 2006;332(7537):339-42.
89. Krumholz A, Wiebe S, Gronseth GS, Gloss DS, Sanchez AM, Kabir AA, et al. Evidence-based guideline: Management of an unprovoked first seizure in adults: Report of the Guideline Development Subcommittee of the American Academy of Neurology and the American Epilepsy Society. Neurology. 2015;84(16):1705-13.
90. Jiménez-Villegas MJ, Lozano-García L, Carrizosa-Moog J. Update on first unprovoked seizure in children and adults: A narrative review. Seizure. 2021;90:28-33.
91. Appendix A: Summary of Evidence-Based Guideline for Clinicians: Management of an Unprovoked First Seizure in Adults. Continuum (Minneap Minn). 2016;22(1 Epilepsy):281-2.
92. Barbosa RMG, Soares MC, Portela DMMC, Guimarães TG, Cury RG. New Perspectives of Deep Brain Stimulation Indications for Parkinson's Disease: A Critical Review. Brain Sci. 2024;14(7):638.
93. Sharma VD, Patel M, Miocinovic S. Surgical Treatment of Parkinson's Disease: Devices and Lesion Approaches. Neurotherapeutics. 2020;17(4):1525-38.
94. Day GS. Rapidly Progressive Dementia. Continuum (Minneap Minn). 2022;28(3):901-36.
95. Hermann P, Zerr I. Rapidly progressive dementias—aetiologies, diagnosis, and management. Nat Rev Neurol. 2022;18:363-76.

SECTION 2

Neuro Muscular

Section Editors: Satish Khadilkar, Achal Kumar Srivastava
Associate Editors: Ayush Agarwal, Abhijeet Gadhave

Q1. How will you approach a patient with neuromuscular weakness?

Ans. A comprehensive history and detailed neuromuscular examination are important initial steps in approaching a patient with neuromuscular weakness. Localizing a lesion in a patient with neuromuscular weakness involves a systematic approach based on clinical features and diagnostic studies. History and examination help differentiate between central and peripheral causes **(Tables 1 and 2)**. In lower motor neuron (LMN) weakness, further localization depends on the pattern of involvement: Anterior horn cell diseases (e.g., motor neuron disease) present with asymmetric weakness, fasciculations, and no sensory loss; nerve root or plexus lesions cause radicular pain or regional weakness; peripheral neuropathies cause distal symmetric weakness with sensory loss; neuromuscular junction disorders [e.g., myasthenia gravis (MG)] exhibit fatigable weakness and cranial muscles involvement without sensory deficits; and myopathies primarily result in a largely symmetric proximal weakness. The following points should be taken into consideration while dealing with a case of neuromuscular weakness **(Tables 3 and 4)**.[1]

TABLE 1: Points in a neuromuscular history.

History Onset	**Acute, subacute, or chronic**
Pattern	Proximal vs. distal weakness, symmetric vs. asymmetric
Progression	Static, progressive, or fluctuating weakness
Associated symptoms	Fatigue, myalgia, cramps, sensory changes, autonomic dysfunction, bulbar symptoms
Triggers	Infection, exercise, medications, and toxins
Family history	Inherited disorders such as muscular dystrophies
Systemic illnesses	Diabetes mellitus, thyroid disorders, malignancy, and autoimmune diseases

TABLE 2: Clinical examination.

Clinical examination	
Inspection	Muscle bulk (atrophy/hypertrophy), fasciculations, any deformities
Power testing	Grading strength using MRC (Medical Research Council) scale
Pattern of weakness	Proximal (myopathy, myasthenia gravis) and distal (neuropathy)
Reflexes	Reduced/absent in peripheral neuropathy
Sensory loss	Suggests neuropathy or a radiculopathy
Cranial nerve involvement	Guillain–Barré syndrome, myasthenia gravis, motor neuron disease, etc.
Autonomic signs	Guillain–Barré syndrome, Lambert–Eaton myasthenic syndrome, etc.

TABLE 3: Diagnostic workup.

Diagnostic workup	
Laboratory tests	Creatine kinase (CK)—myopathies • Antibodies—myasthenia gravis [acetylcholine receptor (AChR) and muscle-specific kinase (MuSK)], autoimmune neuropathies (e.g., ganglioside antibodies, Neurofascin 186, 140, 155) • Thyroid function tests, B12 levels, HbA1c, and metabolic causes
Electrodiagnostic studies	• Nerve conduction studies (NCSs)—neuropathy • Electromyography (EMG)—myopathy, anterior horn cell disease
Imaging	• MRI of brain/spine—central lesions • Muscle imaging—structural abnormalities • MR neurography—nerve root thickening [Guillain–Barré syndrome (GBS) and chronic inflammatory demyelinating polyneuropathy (CIDP)]
Genetic testing	• For inherited neuropathies/myopathies
Other tests	• Lumbar puncture—albuminocytological dissociation • Repetitive nerve stimulation—neuromuscular junction disorders • Muscle biopsy—myositis/dystrophies

TABLE 4: Management of a patient with neuromuscular weakness.

Management	
Supportive care	Symptom relief, physiotherapy, and respiratory support if needed
Specific treatments	• Autoimmune: Immunosuppressants, plasma exchange, and intravenous immunoglobulin (IVIg) • Infections: Antibiotics/antivirals • Genetic: Supportive therapy and gene therapy
Referral	Multidisciplinary care involving neurology, rehabilitation, and allied specialists

Q2. How do you grade myasthenia gravis, and what is the clinical significance of this grading?

Ans. The following clinical parameters have been included in the quantitative myasthenia gravis (QMG) score **(Box 1)**.

Clinical grading is useful for estimating MG weakness and assessing changes in clinical status before and after treatment. The QMG score is simple to use, objective, and can be performed at the bedside.[1]

Q3. Which diagnostic modalities are available for myasthenia gravis?

Ans. The diagnosis of MG is suspected based on weakness of eyelids, external ocular movements, and muscles of chewing and swallowing, along with fatigability and diurnal variation. Diagnosis can be confirmed by performing the following tests **(Flowchart 1)**:

- *Serology*: Serology is the first diagnostic step for MG. *Acetylcholine receptor (AChR)-binding antibodies* are most specific for autoimmune MG. They are found in 80% of patients with generalized MG and 50% with ocular MG. False positive results are rare. Few patients seronegative at the time of diagnosis may seroconvert after 6 months. *Antistriational antibodies* are found in patients of adult-onset MG and patients with thymoma without MG. Muscle-specific *kinase (MuSK) antibodies* are seen in 50% of AChR antibody-negative MG. These patients have the following characteristics:
    - Female preponderance (85%)
    - Predominant facial, pharyngeal, tongue, and respiratory weakness
    - Tongue weakness and furrowing
    - The thymus is normal, thymectomy is not required.
    - Poor prognosis

  In double-seronegative patients (negative for both AChR and MuSK), autoantibodies against *low-density lipoprotein receptor-related protein 4 (LRP-4)* should be tested. Antibody testing is used for diagnostic purposes only and not for clinical follow-up.

BOX 1: Quantitative myasthenia gravis score.

- Double vision on lateral gaze for 60 seconds
- Ptosis on up gaze holding for 60 seconds
- Eyelid closure
- Swallowing half a cup of water
- Speech after counting aloud from 1 to 50
- Both arms outstretched at 90° for 240 seconds
- Forced vital capacity
- Bilateral handgrip for 45 seconds
- Head lifted at 45° for 120 seconds
- Both legs outstretched at 45–50° in the supine position for 100 seconds

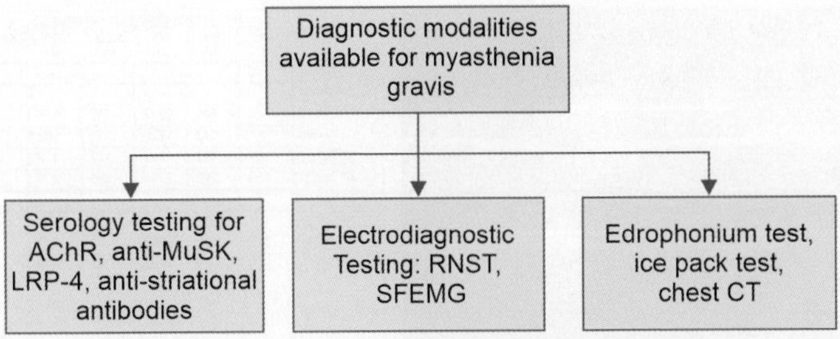

FLOWCHART 1: Diagnostic modalities available for myasthenia gravis.

(AChR: acetylcholine receptor; CT: computed tomography; LRP-4: lipoprotein receptor-related protein 4; MuSK: muscle-specific kinase; RNST: repetitive nerve stimulation testing; SFEMG: single-fiber electromyography)

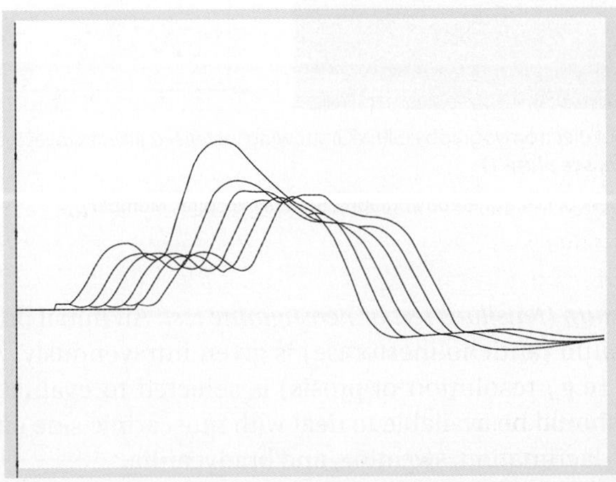

At rest	1.5	–40.1
10-second exercise	1.5	–18.8
1 minute post exercise	0.9	–41.5
2-minute post exercise	0.8	–53.7

FIG. 1: Repetitive nerve stimulation testing (RNST) showing decremental response in myasthenia gravis (MG).

Courtesy: Department of Electroneuromyography, Bombay Hospital, Mumbai.

- *Electrodiagnostic testing*:
  - 2-Hz to 5-Hz repetitive nerve stimulation study shows a compound muscle action potential (CMAP) decrement of >10% **(Fig. 1)**.
  - Single-fiber EMG **(Fig. 2)** is MG's most sensitive diagnostic test. The extensor digitorum communis muscle is studied first. If it is normal, a facial muscle (frontalis/orbicularis oculi) is tested. While single-fiber EMG is sensitive, it is not specific for MG and should not be used in isolation.

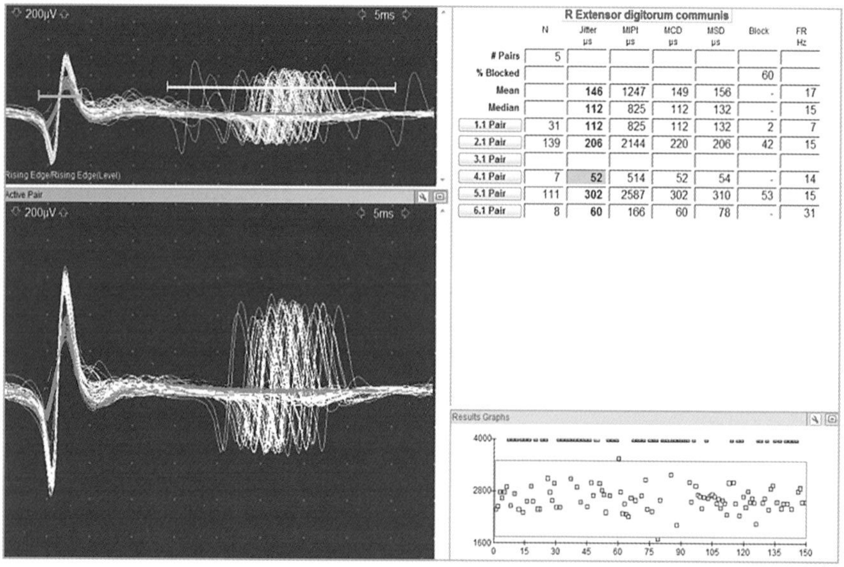

FIG. 2: Single-fiber electromyography (SFEMG) showing increased jitter in myasthenia gravis (MG). ***(For color version, see plate 1)***

Courtesy: Department of Electroneuromyography, Bombay Hospital, Mumbai.

- *Edrophonium (tensilon) test or neostigmine test*: An initial dose of 2 mg of edrophonium (anticholinesterase) is given intravenously. An objective endpoint (e.g., resolution of ptosis) is selected to evaluate the effect. Atropine should be available to deal with muscarinic side effects such as salivation, lacrimation, sweating, and bradycardia.

  When edrophonium is unavailable, injection neostigmine 0.5–2 mg intramuscularly can be given after atropine, and the effects are observed over the next 30–45 minutes.
- *The icepack test*: An ice pack is applied to the weak eyelid for 5 minutes, which results in an improvement of the size of the palpebral fissure by at least 2 mm.
- *Chest CT scan*: It should be performed in patients having MG to rule out thymoma or thymoma recurrence.[2]

Q4. What are available medical treatments for myasthenia gravis?

Ans. The goal in the management of MG is to achieve remission with the least possible side effects from medications. Following medical therapies are available for treatment of MG:

- *Pyridostigmine* is the acetylcholinesterase inhibitor of choice for the symptomatic treatment of MG. Its effect starts within 30–60 minutes and lasts for 3–4 hours. It should be given 30 minutes before meals if dysphagia is the targeted symptom.

- *Corticosteroids* are the first choice for patients of MG because of the rapid onset effect. The initial dose of prednisone should be low (15–20 mg/day) because of a possible risk of short-term exacerbation, especially in bulbar weakness.
- *Mycophenolate mofetil (2–3 g/day) and azathioprine (2–3 mg/kg/day)* are commonly used steroid-sparing agents. Mycophenolate mofetil inhibits monophosphate dehydrogenase, whereas azathioprine blocks nucleotide synthesis. Complete blood count and liver enzymes need to be monitored. For full therapeutic effect, it takes 4–8 months with azathioprine and a few weeks to 2 months with mycophenolate mofetil.
- Intravenous immunoglobulin *(IVIg) (1–2 g/kg over 2–5 days) and plasma exchange (PE) (5–6 exchanges)* are used in generalized MG as a rapid onset, short-term immunomodulation (rescue agents).
- *Rituximab*, a CD20 monoclonal antibody, is used in severe and refractory generalized MG, particularly in MuSK-positive patients.
- *Tacrolimus and cyclosporine* are beneficial for reducing disease burden in both steroid-dependent and new cases. Tacrolimus produces rapid improvement in patients with anti-RyR antibodies.
- *Cyclophosphamide* intravenously has shown benefit in patients with poor disease control on steroids or steroid-sparing agents such as mycophenolate mofetil and azathioprine.
- *Eculizumab* is a complement inhibitor (C5) used in adult patients with AchR-positive generalized MG. To prevent meningococcal infection, patients should be vaccinated before using this drug.[3]

Q5. How would you approach the management of a myasthenic crisis?

Ans. A myasthenic crisis is a true neurological emergency that should be recognized promptly and managed in the ICU with ventilatory support. It is characterized by severe weakness of the diaphragm and accessory respiratory muscles leading to respiratory failure. The most reliable sign of impending respiratory failure is a paradoxical breathing pattern. The single breath count (SBC) is a useful bedside measurement of respiratory function that correlates with vital capacity (VC) and negative inspiratory force (NIF). Several factors have been identified as precipitants of myasthenic crisis as listed here.

- Infections (most common being respiratory infections)
- Medications such as aminoglycosides, procainamide, lignocaine, phenytoin, lithium, barbiturates, and suxamethonium
- Recent trauma and surgery
- Vaccination
- Immune checkpoint inhibitors such as pembrolizumab and nivolumab
- Pregnancy/postpartum
- Botulinum toxin administration

Acute management of myasthenic crisis requires comprehensive care with special attention to ventilatory support. Offending trigger(s) should be identified and removed. IVIg or PE can be used as a rescue therapy as shown in **Flowchart 2.**[4]

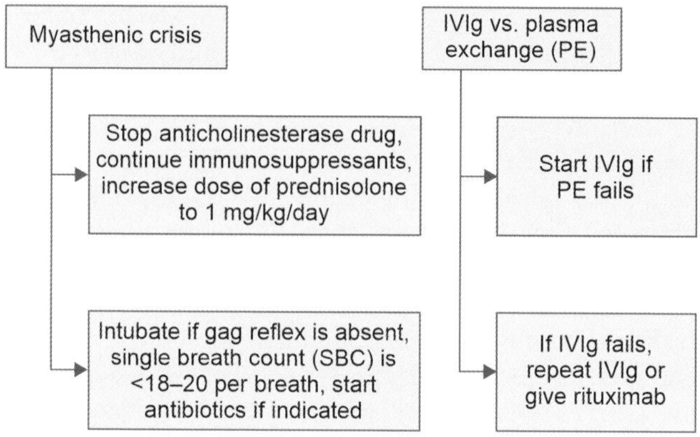

FLOWCHART 2: Treatment protocol in myasthenic crisis.
(IVIg: intravenous immunoglobulin)

Q6. What is refractory myasthenia gravis, and how do you treat it?

Ans. Refractory MG is defined as unchanged or worsening symptoms after treatment with *corticosteroid and at least two other immunosuppressants* used at adequate doses for a significant duration or until adverse side effects occur. Patients with refractory MG frequently experience acute exacerbations of their symptoms. They also have a severely compromised quality of life. The clinical and immunological characteristics associated with refractory MG indicate that there are immunopathological and biological pathways involved in the development of drug-refractory MG. The anti-CD20 monoclonal antibody, rituximab has proven to be highly effective in treating refractory MG, particularly in anti-MuSK positive patients. The terminal complement activation inhibitor eculizumab can be used in such cases. Other options available are cyclophosphamide and thymectomy. A single case report showed improvement in symptoms with bone marrow transplantation in refractory MG.[5]

Q7. What are the indications for thymectomy in patients with myasthenia gravis?

Ans. The thymus plays an important role in the pathogenesis of MG. Approximately 10% of patients with autoimmune MG have a thymoma and 65% of patients have thymic hyperplasia. The preferred surgical approach for thymectomy is a transthoracic, sternal-splitting procedure, which permits wide exploration of the anterior mediastinum. Transcervical, endoscopic approaches and video-assisted thoracoscopic thymectomy (VAT-T) have less postoperative morbidity and short recovery time. Indications for thymectomy in MG are listed here.

- *Thymoma MG*: Thymectomy should be done in all such cases. It has shown benefits in early-onset cases.

- *Early onset MG*: A randomized controlled trial in patients with nonthymomatous MG has shown a significant reduction in steroid dosage and need for multiple immunomodulators. Fewer exacerbation rates were also noted.
- *Late-onset MG*: This group is less responsive to thymectomy. However, it should be considered in patients of age group 50–65 years with severe disease and thymic hyperplasia.
- The presence *of anti-RyR antibodies* indicates that no response will occur after thymectomy.
- *MuSK and LRP 4 MG*: In the absence of thymic pathology, thymectomy is not recommended in this group of patients.
- *Ocular and seronegative MG*: Thymectomy has no role in this group of patients.[6]

Q8. What is Lambert–Eaton myasthenic syndrome (LEMS)?

Ans. Lambert–Eaton myasthenic syndrome is an autoimmune disorder caused by autoantibodies against the P/Q type voltage-gated calcium channels (VGCCs) on presynaptic cholinergic nerve terminals at the neuromuscular junction and autonomic ganglia. This results in the inhibition of Ach release. It was first described in patients with lung cancer. Clinically, patients present with gradual onset proximal lower limb weakness, which progresses and involves proximal upper limbs. Autonomic dysfunction in the form of dry mouth, erectile dysfunction, postural hypotension, constipation, and blurred vision due to pupillary paralysis and dry eyes can be seen. Ocular and bulbar symptoms are less common. Patients also complain of constant muscle fatigue and reduced motor endurance. Hyporeflexia or areflexia with postexercise facilitation is seen in almost 90–100% of patients. Small cell lung carcinoma (SCLC) accounts for 90% of tumors in patients with tumor-associated LEMS (T-LEMS). DELTA-P score is used to predict the presence of SCLC in a patient with LEMS **(Table 5)**. The classical electrophysiological findings of LEMS are a low CMAP at rest, a decremental response to low-rate stimulation, and an incremental response to high-rate stimulation **(Fig. 3)**. Apart from P/Q type VGCC antibodies, other serological markers seen in LEMS are SOX1, muscarinic AChRs, and synaptotagmin. Screening for tumors, especially SCLC, should be done in all patients. Initially, a CT thorax should be done and if negative, a positron emission tomography (PET) scan of the whole body should be done. Symptomatic therapy (3,4-Diaminopyridine) helps to deal with decreased Ach in synaptic terminals by blocking presynaptic voltage-gated potassium channels. IVIg and PE can be used as a rescue therapy for rapid worsening of the muscle strength. Oral steroids and steroid-sparing agents (mycophenolate mofetil and azathioprine) can be used for long-term management. It is important to screen for SCLC and start appropriate antitumor therapy.[7]

TABLE 5: DELTA-P scoring system.

	Categories	Within 3 months of onset	Score
D	Dysarthria, dysphagia, chewing, neck weakness: Bulbar weakness	Absent	0
		Present	1
E	Erectile dysfunction	Female	0
		Male: Absent	0
		Male: Present	1
L	Loss of weight	Absent or <5%	0
		≥5%	1
T	Tobacco use at onset	Absent	0
		Present	1
A	Age of onset	<50 years	0
		≥50 years	1
P	Karnofsky performance score	70–100	0
		0–60	1

Motor NCS

Nerve	Sites	Amp. 2–4 mV	Lat. ms	Amp. 1–2 mV	Area%	Dur.%	Dur. ms
R median-APB	1. Wrist	1.6	4.50	1.1	100	100	5.20
	2. Post 10 seconds ex	10.0	4.00	6.9	648	121	6.30

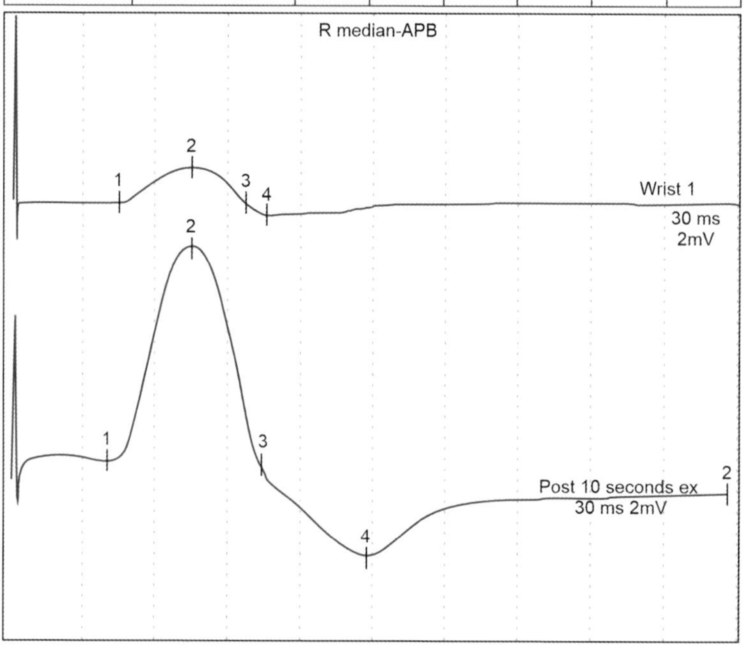

FIG. 3: Short exercise test in LEMS: Low amplitude baseline CMAP in trace 1; immediately following a 10-second exercise, the CMAP improves by 100%.

(CMAP: compound muscle action potential; LEMS: Lambert–Eaton myasthenic syndrome)

Courtesy: Department of Electroneuromyography, Bombay Hospital, Mumbai.

Q9. How do inflammatory myopathies present?

Ans. Inflammatory myopathies include dermatomyositis, immune-mediated necrotizing myopathy, inclusion body myositis, antisynthetase syndrome, and overlap myositis. Clinical features of inflammatory myopathies are listed here.

- *Muscle weakness in inflammatory myopathies*: Muscle weakness is symmetric and proximal, often involving the proximal shoulder and hip girdle limb muscles. It may progress to involve truncal muscles. Distal muscle weakness occurs late in the disease process. However, early involvement of finger flexors (decreased grip strength) is characteristic of inclusion body myositis **(Fig. 4)**. Ocular muscles are usually spared. Facial muscle weakness is mild. Neck flexor weakness is more common than neck extensor weakness. Involvement of pharyngeal muscles may cause hoarseness of voice, nasal regurgitation, and dysphagia leading to aspiration pneumonia. In advanced cases, the patient may develop diaphragmatic weakness leading to respiratory insufficiency.
- *Dermatomyositis*: Dermatomyositis presents with a subacute onset proximal muscle weakness that accompanies or follows a distinct skin rash. Some patients may develop a rash without any weakness (*dermatomyositis sine myositis or amyopathic dermatomyositis*). A pathognomonic heliotrope (violaceous discoloration) rash is often seen in the upper eyelids **(Fig. 5A)**. The cutaneous manifestations of the rash are seen over the anterior chest (V sign), back, and shoulders (shawl sign). Erythematous eruptions and raised papules on bony prominences, especially metacarpophalangeal, proximal interphalangeal, and distal interphalangeal joints are known as Gottron papules **(Fig. 5B)**. Other features of dermatomyositis include mechanic's hands, telangiectasias, and calcinosis cutis. Extramuscular manifestations include pulmonary, cardiac, gastrointestinal, and joint systems.

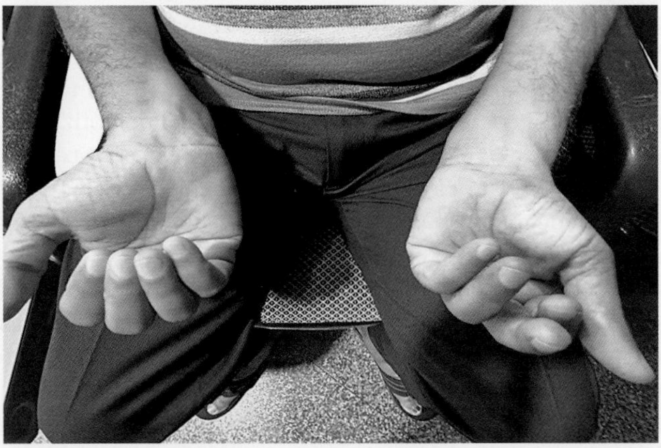

FIG. 4: On attempting to make a fist, the patient cannot fully close the hand due to finger flexor weakness in inclusion body myositis. ***(For color version, see plate 1)***

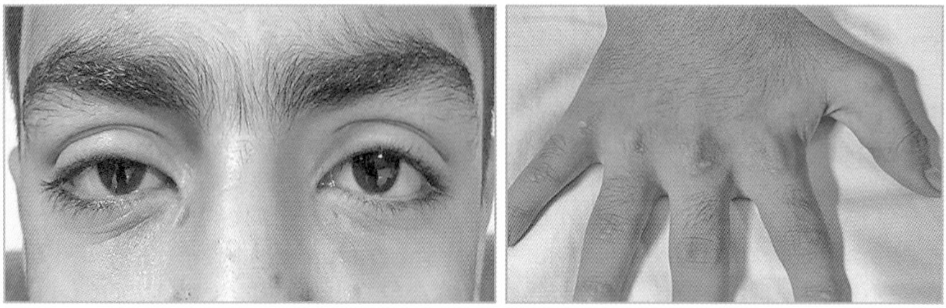

FIGS. 5A AND B: (A) Heliotrope rash; and (B) Gottron papules. ***(For color version, see plate 2)***

- *Antisynthetase syndrome*: Patients may have a constellation of inflammatory myopathy, interstitial lung disease (ILD), arthritis, Raynaud syndrome, fever, skin rash, and mechanic's hands. Muscle weakness is common in patients positive for anti-Jo-1 autoantibodies.
- *Immune-mediated necrotizing myopathies*: They present with severe proximal muscle weakness (acute/subacute). Extramuscular involvement is rare (<10% of cases).
- *Overlap myositis*: Myopathy is associated with other connective tissue disorders such as systemic lupus erythematosus (SLE), Sjögren syndrome, rheumatoid arthritis, and systemic sclerosis.
- *Inclusion body myositis*: They have a slowly progressive preferential pattern of involvement of quadriceps, finger flexors, and ankle dorsiflexors.[8]

Q10. What are the modalities available for the diagnosis of inflammatory myopathies?

Ans. Several diagnostic tools are available for evaluating patients suspected of having inflammatory myopathies. These include serum creatine kinase (CK) and other serum enzymes, electrodiagnostic (EDX) studies, myositis antibodies, muscle biopsy, and muscle MRI.

- *Serum CK and other serum enzymes*: Serum CK levels are often elevated due to muscle membrane damage and necrosis in patients with myositis. In dermatomyositis, they may range from normal to up to thousands of international units per liter. In immune-mediated necrotizing myopathy, CK levels are elevated to several thousands. CK elevation can precede the onset of weakness. Other enzymatic markers elevated include aldolase, lactate dehydrogenase (LDH), aspartate transaminase (AST) and alanine transaminase (ALT).
- *EDX studies*: These can confirm the myopathic processes and can rule out neurogenic causes of proximal muscle weakness such as chronic inflammatory demyelinating polyradiculoneuropathy, and motor neuron disease. In patients with myopathies, sensory and motor nerve conduction studies are normal. EMG shows spontaneous activity (fibrillation potentials and positive sharp waves) and short-duration, low-amplitude motor unit potentials with early recruitment.

- *Histopathology*: The classical feature of dermatomyositis is perifascicular muscle fiber atrophy. The inflammatory infiltrates (CD4+ T cells and plasmacytoid dendritic cells) are located in the perimysium and perivascular region. In antisynthetase syndrome, necrosis in the perifascicular region with increased perimysial alkaline phosphatase activity is seen. On electron microscopy, aggregation of nuclear actin is seen. Inclusion body myositis shows endomysial inflammation and rimmed vacuoles. Proteinaceous inclusions are seen in IBM on histology and electron microscopy.
- *Muscle MRI*: In dermatomyositis, short tau inversion recovery (STIR) images show hyperintensity/edema in patchy distribution in muscle along with subcutaneous tissue and fascia. It also helps detect calcinosis deposits. Two distinct features of immune-mediated necrotizing myopathy are minimal fascial edema and less involvement of the anterior compartment of the thigh. Muscle MRIs of patients with anti-signal recognition particle (SRP) myopathy show higher rates of fatty replacement and atrophy.[9]

Myositis antibodies are shown in **Table 6**.

TABLE 6: Myositis antibodies and associated clinical features.

Myositis antibodies	Clinical features
Dermatomyositis	
Anti-Mi-2	Skin rash, muscle involvement, and good response to immunotherapy
Anti-TIF-1	Strong association with cancer
Anti-NXP-2	Associated with malignancy, subcutaneous calcifications, mild-to-moderate muscle involvement
Anti-MDA-5	Rapidly progressive interstitial lung disease (ILD), severe skin rash, and mild muscle involvement
Anti-SAE	Rash, dysphagia, and muscle involvement
Antisynthetase syndrome	
Anti-JO-1	Muscle involvement, ILD, skin rash, and mechanic's hands
Anti-PL-7	Severe ILD, moderate muscle involvement
Anti-PL-12	Severe ILD, mild or no muscle involvement
Anti-glycyl-transfer RNA synthetase	ILD
Immune-mediated necrotizing myopathy	
Anti-signal recognition particle (SRP)	Severe muscle involvement
Anti-3-hydroxy-3-methylglutaryl coenzyme A (HMG-CoA) reductase	Severe muscle involvement, history of statin use
Antibody-negative immune-mediated necrotizing myopathy	Increased risk of malignancy

Q11. What are the medical treatments for inflammatory myopathies?

Ans. Standardized consensus guidelines for the treatment of inflammatory myopathies do not exist. Treatment is mainly based on case series and the opinions of experts. Following are the various treatment modalities available for inflammatory myopathies.

- *Corticosteroids:* They are first-line therapy in the treatment of inflammatory myopathies. Prednisone is prescribed at a dose of 0.5 mg/kg/day to 1 mg/kg/day (maximum dose of 60–80 mg/day). In severe cases, intravenous methylprednisolone can be given initially. A very slow rate of taper is advised to prevent disease flare-ups. Long-term side effects of steroids such as hypertension, weight gain, osteoporosis, and deranged blood glucose levels need to be monitored. A second immunosuppressive steroid-sparing agent should be started early in moderate-to-severe cases.
- *Steroid-sparing immunosuppressants*: These include methotrexate (10–20 mg/week orally or subcutaneously), azathioprine (2–3 mg/kg/day), mycophenolate mofetil (2–3 g/day divided into two daily doses), or maintenance IVIg (1 g/kg/month administered over 2–3 days).
- *IVIg:* It can be effective in refractory dermatomyositis, and immune-mediated necrotizing myopathy, particularly in patients with anti-HMG-CoA reductase antibodies.
- *Rituximab (anti-CD20 monoclonal antibody)*: It is effective in refractory inflammatory myopathy, patients with antisynthetase syndrome (anti-Jo-1), anti-Mi-2 antibody positive cases, and patients with anti-SRP antibody immune-mediated necrotizing myopathy who are refractory to conventional immunotherapies.
- *Calcineurin inhibitors:* Cyclosporine and tacrolimus should be used with caution owing to their renal toxicity.
- *Cyclophosphamide:* It can be used in refractory cases, in patients who have rapidly progressive interstitial lung disease but can cause infertility.
- *Biologic agents:* Newer biological agents include antitumor necrosis factor agents (etanercept and infliximab), anti-interleukin 6 (IL6) (tocilizumab), anti-CD52 monoclonal antibody (alemtuzumab), anti-interferon-alpha monoclonal antibody (sifalimumab), a monoclonal antibody blocking IL2 receptor alpha-chain, and CD25 antigen (basiliximab).[10]

Q12. What is the clinical spectrum of common limb-girdle muscular dystrophy seen in India?

Ans. Limb-girdle muscular dystrophy (LGMDs) are a group of genetic myopathies that present as chronic progressive weakness of hip and shoulder girdles. The clinical spectrum of common LGMDs is described here.

- *Prominent upper girdle involvement:* Scapular winging **(Fig. 6)** without facial weakness is commonly seen in calpainopathy. It is also seen in sarcoglycanopathies, fukutin-related proteinopathy, and anoctaminopathy. "Calf head on trophy sign" is seen in dysferlinopathy. Early and prominent facial involvement **(Fig. 7)** favors facioscapulohumeral muscular dystrophy.

- *Biceps lump and diamond on quadriceps' sign:* Biceps lump **(Fig. 8)** results from partial hypertrophy of the biceps muscle and wasting of the remaining part of the muscle. The combination of atrophy with hypertrophy of the quadriceps muscle leads to a diamond-like configuration **(Fig. 9)** on the thigh. Both are seen in dysferlinopathy.

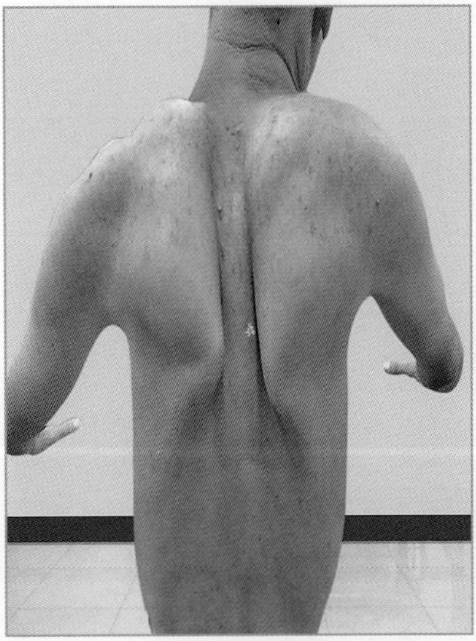

FIG. 6: Scapular winging in calpainopathy. ***(For color version, see plate 2)***

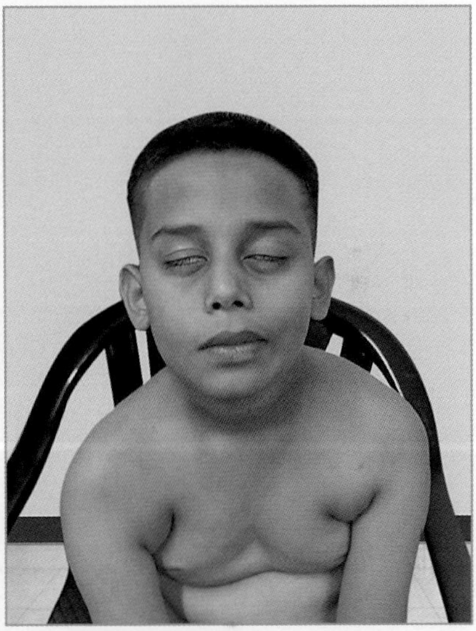

FIG. 7: Early facial involvement is seen in facioscapulohumeral muscular dystrophy (FSHD). ***(For color version, see plate 2)***

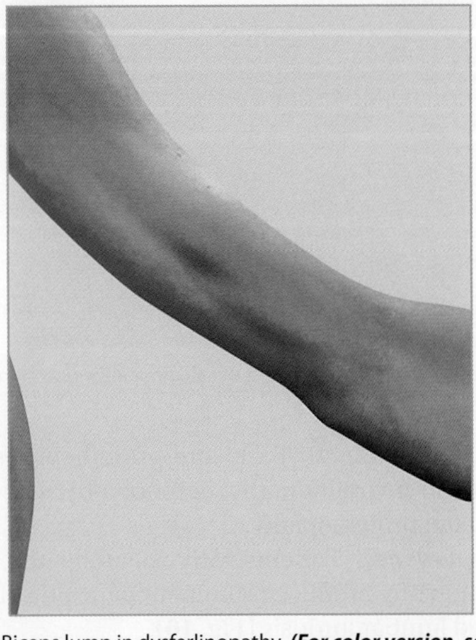

FIG. 8: Biceps lump in dysferlinopathy. ***(For color version, see plate 3)***

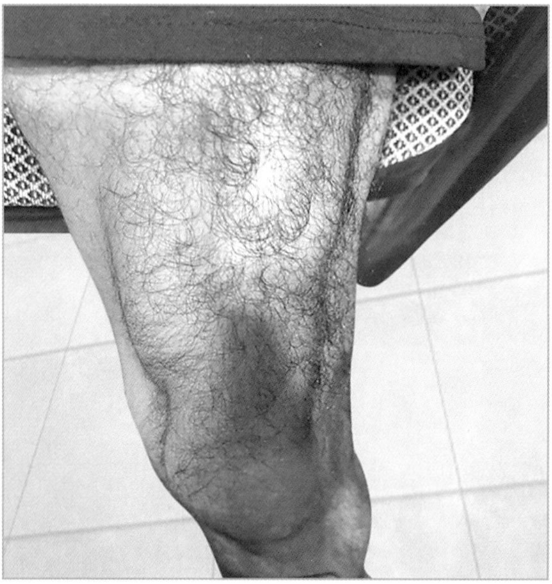

FIG. 9: Diamond on quadriceps in dysferlinopathy. ***(For color version, see plate 3)***

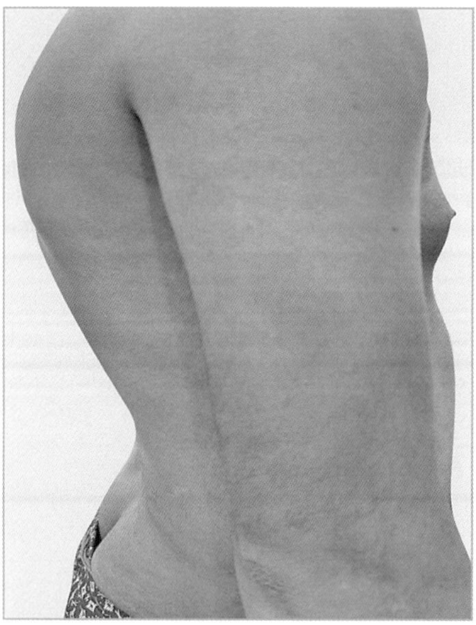

FIG. 10: Exaggerated lumbar lordosis in a patient of calpainopathy. ***(For color version, see plate 4)***

- *Respiratory muscle weakness:* Early and prominent respiratory muscle weakness occurs in myotilinopathy, laminopathy, sarcoglycanopathies, and fukutin-related proteinopathy.
- *Truncal muscle weakness:* Patients with calpainopathy, dysferlinopathy, and sarcoglycanopathy produce prominent paraspinal muscle weakness with exaggerated lumbar lordosis **(Fig. 10)**.

- *Abdominal muscle weakness:* Calpainopathy patients develop abdominal muscle weakness, prominent visceroptosis, and herniation of abdominal organs.
- *Hip abduction sign:* Some patients with LGMDs have disproportionately weak hip adductors. There is abduction of thighs when the patient attempts to get up from the ground. This sign was initially described in sarcoglycanopathies and is also seen in calpainopathies.
- *Prominent distal weakness:* Patients with anterior leg compartment weakness (tibialis anterior) produce a foot drop **(Fig. 11)** seen in GNE myopathy, myotilinopathy, desminopathy, telethoninopathy, and titinopathy. Weakness of the posterior compartment of the leg (gastrocnemius and soleus) presents with calf atrophy **(Fig. 12)** and leads to an inability to stand on toes. This is seen in dysferlinopathy and anoctaminopathy.
- *Calf hypertrophy:* Calf hypertrophy **(Fig. 13)** is classically seen in Duchenne and Becker's muscular dystrophy. Calf hypertrophy with proximal muscle weakness in a girl in the first decade points toward autosomal recessive limb girdle muscular dystrophies such as sarcoglycanopathy.
- *Contractures:* Contractures at the ankle joint (leading to toe walking), and elbow joints are common in calpainopathy. Contractures at intervertebral joints causing a rigid spine are common in laminopathy.
- *Cardiac involvement:* It is more common in autosomal-dominant LGMDs than in the recessive types. Dilated and hypertrophic cardiomyopathies are common in sarcoglycanopathy and dystroglycanopathy. Conduction defects are common in laminopathy.[11]

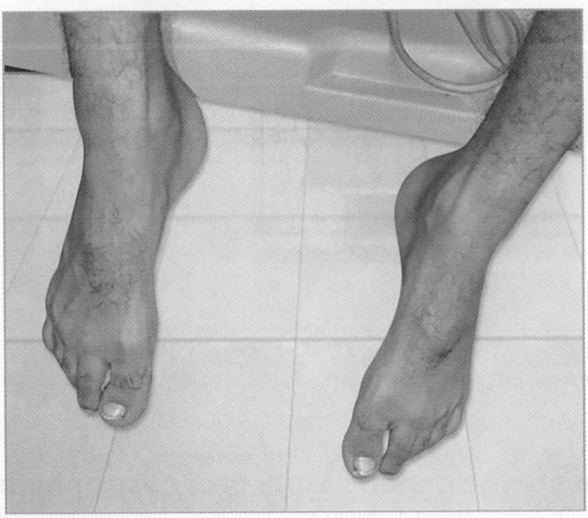

FIG. 11: Foot drop in GNE myopathy. ***(For color version, see plate 4)***

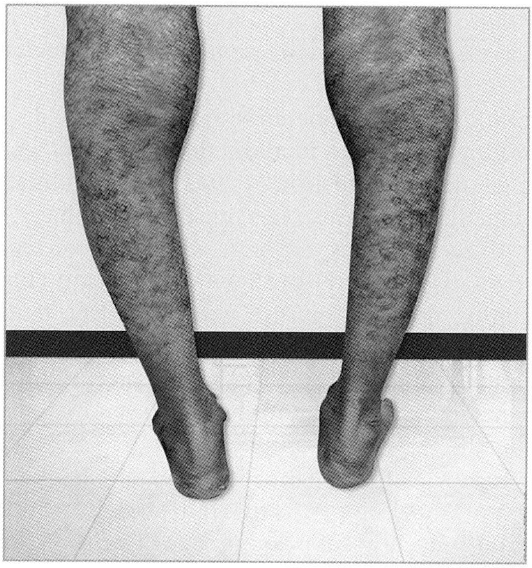

FIG. 12: Calf atrophy in dysferlinopathy. ***(For color version, see plate 5)***

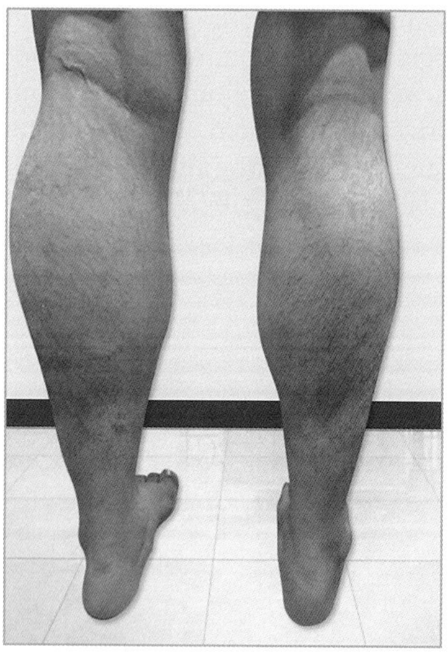

FIG. 13: Calf hypertrophy in Duchenne muscular dystrophy. ***(For color version, see plate 5)***

Q13. What are the genetic aspects of dystrophinopathies?

Ans. Dystrophinopathies, namely the Duchenne muscular dystrophy (DMD) and Becker muscular dystrophy (BMD), are common in clinical practice; hence, it is important to know their genetic basis. These conditions are inherited as X-linked recessive. Hence, usually, the male is the sufferer, as he has only one X. Females are carriers, as they have two X chromosomes. Rarely, can females manifest the disease, in situations such as Turner syndrome, X-autosome translocation, and mosaicism. The genetic defect is located on the short arm of the X chromosome at the locus Xp21. The dystrophin gene is a large gene stretching over 2,000 kilobase pairs and has 79 exons. 70–80% of patients have a deletion of one or more of these 79 exons. There are some hot spots in the gene, meaning that the deletions are more common in these areas of the genes. 10–15% of the patients have a duplication of some of the exons, and the remaining have point mutations. The deletions are detected by multiplex polymerase chain reaction (PCR) test. With the knowledge of the hot spots, the appropriate probes have been prepared and are commercially available for use. These usually test 32 exons that are commonly deleted. Multiplex PCR for the dystrophin gene is now widely available in India and is comparatively inexpensive. This test will detect the common deletions. The next test is the multiple ligation-dependent probe amplification (MLPA). This studies all 79 exons and being a quantitative test, can detect the dosing effect. This test is used to detect duplications in addiction to deletions. The test is also useful for carrier detection for mothers and sisters of affected individuals. Thus, the multiplex PCR and MLPA can detect 85–90% of defects in the dystrophin gene (deletions and duplications). The remaining, point mutations, require new-generation sequencing (NGS). This test can pick out changes in single amino acids.

The type of mutation has a bearing on the phenotype. A mutation can be "in frame" or "out of frame". When the remaining fragments of the gene are such that they can join together, they can produce a smaller version of the gene product, the dystrophin, and the clinical phenotype will be milder, like BMD. This is called the "reading frame hypotheses". The following sentence will elucidate this hypothesis.[12]

You can see the boy (imagine this to be the dystrophin gene)

You see the boy (There is a missing word, but the remaining sentence is meaningful—BMD phenotype)

You ca ee the boy (the remaining sentence is not meaningful—DMD phenotype)

Q14. What are the newer modalities of treatment available for dystrophinopathies?

Ans. Treatment strategies for the management of dystrophinopathies can be divided into two categories: (1) Increasing dystrophin protein expression and (2) altering the effects of pathologic processes. Treatment strategies can either be mutation-specific or mutation-agnostic. Currently, two drugs are approved by the US Food and Drug Administration (FDA) for dystrophinopathy. This includes mutation-specific eteplirsen and mutation-agnostic deflazacort (0.9 mg/kg/day). The exon-51-skipping therapy (eteplirsen) uses antisense oligonucleotides to restore the reading frame by "skipping" and exon. Deflazacort can be used in all patients with severe

TABLE 7: List of drugs in development for Duchenne muscular dystrophy (DMD) with their mechanism of action.

Drugs in development	Mechanism of action
Mini-dystrophin, micro-dystrophin	Gene transfer
Eteplirsen, multi-exon skipping (in development)	Exon skipping
Ataluren	A read-through of a premature termination codon
Muscle growth drugs	Human anti-myostatin antibody, follistatin
Selective androgen receptor modulator	DT-200
Anti-inflammatory drugs	Prednisolone and deflazacort
Inhibitors of nuclear factor-kappa B	Vamorolone
Antioxidant	Idebenone
Antifibrotics, anti-tumor growth factor beta (TGF-β) drugs	Losartan, halofuginone, and fibrinogen

dystrophinopathy. Ataluren, approved in Europe, works by a read-through of premature termination codon and is used in patients with a DMD nonsense mutation **(Table 7)**.[13]

Q15. What are the clinical cues for myotonic muscular dystrophy?

Ans. Myotonic dystrophy is of two types, DM1 and DM2. DM1 is also called Steinert's disease and four types, classic, mild, congenital, and childhood, are recognized. DM2 is also known as the proximal myotonic myopathy.

The classic form usually presents in early adulthood. Patients develop features of myotonia and dystrophy. Myotonia causes a delay in the relaxation process, hence patients experience difficulty in releasing the handgrip, and some stiffness and slowness of motor activities. In general, myotonic manifestations are not as prominent as in myotonia congenita. The dominant feature in DM1 is weakness and wasting of the muscles. The muscles commonly affected are the small muscles of the hand and as a result, patients have difficulty in doing fine motor tasks with their hands. They can also have difficulty in speaking, chewing, and swallowing, and gait changes. Early fatigue also sets in due to muscular weakness. Cardiac complaints such as palpitations are common due to the effect of the conduction system. The childhood form is similar to the adult form but for early appearance and in the mild form, as the word implies, the symptoms are mild. The congenital form is a very severe form, and children are born hypotonic and have difficulty in sucking and a weak cry. Club feet are seen. The symptoms may begin antenatally, fetal movements tend to be weak, and polyhydramnios may be seen. The clinical signs lead to the diagnosis. Myotonia can be elicited in two ways, the grip and percussion myotonia. When eliciting grip myotonia, ask the patient to grip the examiner's fingers for about 15 seconds and then release the grip. The

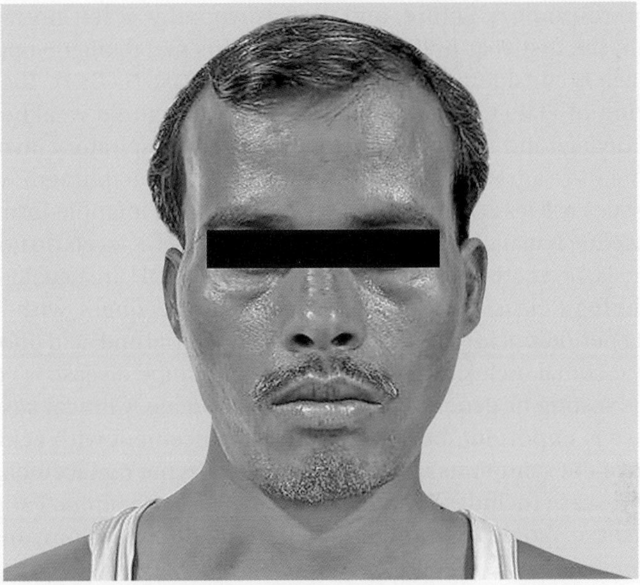

FIG. 14: Hatchet facies, frontal balding, and wasting of the temporalis muscles in myotonic muscular dystrophy. ***(For color version, see plate 5)***

release will be slow. For percussion myotonia, the examiner taps a muscle with the percussion hammer, and the muscle can be seen to contract and then slowly relax. Thenar muscles or the extensors of the wrist can be chosen for this sign. DM1 patients tend to be long and slender face (hatchet face) with wasting of the temporalis and masseter muscles and low-set ears; the angles of the mouth tend to be downturned (fish mouth of bouche de tapir); and the weakness of the sternomastoid muscles gives the appearance of the swan neck. Frontal balding is seen. Patients can have ptosis and sometimes keep their mouths open due to the weakness of their jaw muscles **(Fig. 14)**.

Myotonic dystrophy 1 is a multisystem disorder, and the manifestations go beyond the muscles. Patients can have cardiac conduction defects, cardiac failure, premature cataracts, behavioral and cognitive changes, testicular atrophy, gastrointestinal (GI) symptoms, and there is some increase in the cancer risk.

Myotonic dystrophy 2 is also called the proximal myotonic myopathy. This type is uncommon and presents with proximal weakness of the hip girdle muscles, leading to difficulty in rising from the ground, climbing stairs, and knee buckling. Myotonia may be subtle.[14]

Q16. What are the clinical features, diagnostics, and therapeutics of Pompe disease?

Ans. Pompe disease, or glycogen storage disorder (GSD2), is an autosomal recessive disease, resulting from mutations in the *GAA* gene. This leads to an enzymatic deficiency of acid maltase. The incidence of Pompe disease is 1 in 9,000 to 1 in 40,000 people. The infantile form presents with profound myopathy, respiratory failure, and cardiomyopathy; if left untreated it is fatal within the first year of life. The onset of this metabolic myopathy after 1 year of age is considered late-onset Pompe disease (LOPD). The classical presentation of LOPD is a slowly progressive limb-girdle weakness that is worse in the legs and axial musculature with early respiratory involvement. The decline in respiratory function is mainly due to diaphragm weakness. Cardiac issues are less common in LOPD than in the infantile form. The CK level at baseline is usually elevated. However, normal CK levels do not rule out the diagnosis. Liver enzymes such as ALT, AST, and LDH are usually elevated. Histopathology classically demonstrated muscle fibers with vacuoles containing periodic acid–Schiff (PAS) positive material and acid phosphatase positive lysosomal inclusions. The diagnosis of Pompe disease is confirmed by enzyme testing or genetic sequencing of the gene. Clinical suspicion of this disease is important, because enzyme replacement with acid maltase can improve the symptoms of illness. Specific enzyme replacement therapy in Pompe disease includes IV infusion of alglucosidase alpha. Patients with Pompe disease should be monitored and treated for cardiomyopathy and conduction defects.[14]

Q17. How will you differentiate between neuropathies based on their clinical course?

Ans. Table 8 differentiates between neuropathies based on their clinical course.[15]

Q18. What scoring system is used to grade muscle strength in neuromuscular disorders at diagnosis and follow up?[16]

Ans. *MRC (Medical Research Council) sum score.*[16]

TABLE 8: Difference between neuropathies based on their clinical course.

Acute onset (days)	Subacute onset (weeks to months)	Chronic onset/ insidious onset	Relapsing remitting course
GBS	Toxin/Medication associated	CIDP	GBS
Acute intermittent porphyria	Nutritional/ Metabolic deficiency	Hereditary motor sensory neuropathies	CIDP
Diphtheric neuropathy	Paraneoplastic	Pure sensory neuropathies	HIV/AIDS
Thallium toxicity	CIDP		Toxic
Critical illness neuropathy	Infectious		Porphyria

(AIDS: acquired immunodeficiency syndrome; CIDP: chronic inflammatory demyelinating polyneuropathy; GBS: Guillain–Barré syndrome; HIV: human immunodeficiency virus)

This score is the sum of MRC scores from 6 muscles in the upper and lower limbs on both sides. It ranges between 60 (normal) and 0 (quadriplegic) **(Table 9)**.

Q19. What are prediction models for respiratory insufficiency available for severe Guillain–Barré syndrome?

Ans. Erasmus GBS Respiratory Insufficiency Score (EGRIS) is the major prediction model for respiratory insufficiency in Guillain-Barré syndrome (GBS). Higher scores are associated with greater chances of requirement of mechanical ventilation **(Table 10)**.[17]

TABLE 9: MRC (Medical Research Council) sum score.

Muscle		Score	MRC scale for muscle strength (0–5)
Shoulder abductors	Right		• Grade 0—no visible contraction • Grade 1—visible contraction without movement of the limb • Grade 2—movement of the limb but not against gravity • Grade 3—movement against gravity but not against resistance • Grade 4—movement against gravity and resistance • Grade 5—normal
	Left		
Elbow flexors	Right		
	Left		
Wrist extensors	Right		
	Left		
Hip abductors	Right		
	Left		
Knee extensors	Right		
	Left		
Ankle dorsiflexors	Right		
	Left		

TABLE 10: Erasmus GBS Respiratory Insufficiency Score (EGRIS).

Measure	Categories	Score
Days between onset of weakness and hospital admission	>7 days	0
	4–7 days	1
	≤3 days	2
Facial and/or bulbar weakness at admission	Presence	1
	Absence	0
MRC sum score at hospital admission	51–60	0
	41–50	1
	31–40	2
	21–30	3
	≤20	4
		0–7

(MRC: Medical Research Council)

Q20. What is the diagnostic criteria for diagnosing Guillain–Barré syndrome?

Ans. Guillain–Barré syndrome is diagnosed based on the *modified Asbury criteria*. The criteria are:

Features required for the diagnosis:
- Progressive bilateral weakness of arms and legs (initially only legs may be involved)
- Absent or decreased deep tendon reflexes in the affected limbs

Features strongly supportive of the diagnosis:
- Progressive phase lasts from days up to 4 weeks (usually <2 weeks)
- Relatively symmetrical signs and symptoms
- Relatively mild sensory signs and symptoms (or absent)
- Cranial nerve involvement (especially bilateral facial palsy)
- Autonomic dysfunction
- Muscular/radicular/limb pain
- Increased protein in the cerebrospinal fluid (normal protein level does not rule out)
- Electrodiagnostic features of motor or sensorimotor neuropathy (normal findings early in the disease course do not rule out the diagnosis)

Red flags:
- Increased mononuclear or polymorphonuclear cells in cerebrospinal fluid (CSF) ($>50 \times 10^6$/L)
- Marked, persistent asymmetrical weakness
- Bowel or bladder impairment at onset or persistent during the disease
- Severe respiratory involvement with limited limb weakness at onset
- Fever at onset
- Nadir < 24 hours
- Sharp sensory level
- Hyper-reflexia or clonus
- Extensor plantar response
- Abdominal pain
- Symptom progression >4 weeks after symptom onset
- Alteration in level of consciousness[18,19]

Q21. What are available medical treatments for Guillain–Barré syndrome?

Ans. Patients with GBS can either be treated with intravenous immunoglobulin (IVIg) or plasmapheresis (PLEX). IVIg is transfused at a total dose of 2 g/kg body weight (divided over 5 days) and PLEX is conducted over five sessions on alternate days exchanging 200–250 mL plasma/kg body weight. Both are equally efficacious.

Both treatments can be safely used in pregnant patients (IVIg preferred) and children.

Plasmapheresis followed by IVIg and repeat IVIg dosing has not proven more effective than either treatment alone.

Corticosteroid treatment has not shown any benefit in multiple randomized controlled trials. Oral corticosteroid treatment was even shown to have an adverse effect on outcome.

No other treatment has proven to be effective in the treatment of GBS.[19]

Q22. What are the common culprits for drug-induced neuropathies?

Ans. Table 11 shows the common culprits for drug-induced neuropathies.[20]

TABLE 11: Common culprits for drug-induced neuropathies.

Drug	Dosage	Risk factors	Pathogenesis	DIPN type
Cardiovascular agent-related DIPN				
Statins	No specific dose. Increased treatment duration and cumulative dose associated with increased risk	Treatment duration >2 years	Alterations of membrane function, disruption of ubiquinone synthesis, and energy utilization in nerves	Axonal; primarily sensory neuropathy
Amiodarone	>200 mg dose has highest association	Increased dose and duration of therapy	Demyelination, loss of large axons with lysosomal inclusions; oxidative stress	Demyelinating; sensory motor
Chemotherapeutic agent-related DIPN				
Vinca alkaloids	2 mg	Single and cumulative dose level	Microtubule-mediated cellular and axonal transport dysfunction	Axonal; sensory
Platinum	60 mg/m^2	Single and cumulative dose level, infusion duration, and treatment duration	Chronic (cisplatin and oxaliplatin)—irreversible cross linking to DNA and neuronal apoptosis Acute (oxaliplatin)—voltage-dependent sodium channel dysfunction	Cisplatin—axonal sensory Oxaliplatin—acute symptoms and chronic sensory

Continued

Continued

Drug	Dosage	Risk factors	Pathogenesis	DIPN type
Bortezomib	Fifth cycle dose of 30 mg/ m^2	Single and cumulative dose level, treatment duration	Mitochondrial dysfunction	Axonal; Small fiber sensory
Thalidomide	>200 mg/day	Single and cumulative dose level, treatment duration	Mitochondrial dysfunction	Axonal; sensory
Arsenic trioxide	10 mg/day		Acute axonal damage and demyelination	Chronic sensory and motor
Taxanes	175 mg/m^2 every 3 weeks	Increased frequency and dose; cumulative dose	Interfere with metabolic calcium signaling; disruption of tubulin depolymerization in axonal transport	Axonal; sensory predominant with motor deficits when severe
Antibiotic-related DIPN				
Isoniazid		Alcohol dependence, diabetes, malnutrition, pregnancy, elderly, HIV	Interference with vitamin B6 synthesis	Axonal; sensory
Ethambutol		Increased age, prolonged duration of treatment, higher dose, hypertension, poor renal function, diabetes, alcohol, and tobacco use	Zinc chelation affecting mitochondrial metal-containing enzymes and excitotoxic pathway	Optic neuropathy
Linezolid		Prolonged treatment and increased doses	Unknown; might be related to protein inhibition and mitochondrial dysfunction	Optic neuropathy; axonal sensory
Metroni-dazole		Prolonged treatment and increased doses	Axonal degeneration secondary to binding to neuronal RNA	Optic neuropathy; axonal sensory and motor

Continued

Continued

Drug	Dosage	Risk factors	Pathogenesis	DIPN type
Immunosuppressant-related DIPN				
Biologicals		Dose and duration	T-cell and B-cell immune attack on peripheral myelin; vasculitis-induced nerve ischemia	GBS, Miller Fischer syndrome, CIDP, MMNCB, and vasculitic neuropathy
Leflunomide		Older age, diabetes, previous exposure to neurotoxic drugs, and alcoholism	Drug-induced neurologic vasculitis and epineural perivascular inflammation	Axonal; sensory or sensory motor
Interferons		Concomitant autoimmune disease	Immune-mediated myelin degradation, vasculitis, induction of anti-GM1 antibodies	GBS, CIDP, and vasculitic neuropathy
Other agent-related DIPN				
Levodopa	• Average dose >700 mg/day • Highest risk at dose >1,500 mg/day	High-dose treatment, hyperhomocysteinemia, low vitamin B12, and low BMI	Accumulation of serum homocysteine and cobalamin-related metabolites, free radical accumulation	Axonal; sensory
NRTIs	• Zalcitabine: 2.25 mg/day • Didanosine: 400 mg/day • Lamivudine: 300 mg/day	Prior neuropathy, underlying malignancy, low CD4 count, high dose, combination therapy, alcohol use, and metabolic impairments	Inhibition of gamma-DNA polymerase leading to mitochondrial dysfunction	Axonal; sensory

(BMI: body mass index; CIDP: chronic inflammatory demyelinating polyneuropathy; DIPN: drug-induced peripheral neuropathy; GBS: Guillain–Barré syndrome; HIV: human immunodeficiency virus; MMNCB: multifocal motor neuropathy with conduction block)

Q23. What are the diagnostic criteria for chronic inflammatory demyelinating polyneuropathy?

Ans. Table 12 shows the diagnostic criteria for CIDP.[21]

TABLE 12: EFNS/PNS 2021 diagnostic criteria for CIDP.

Clinical criteria	Typical	Atypical
	Chronically progressive, stepwise or recurrent symmetric proximal and distal weakness and sensory dysfunction in all extremities that developed over ≥2 months with absent or reduced tendon reflexes in all extremities	DADS
		MADSAM
		Focal (brachial or lumbosacral)
		Pure motor
		Pure sensory
	• *Not* caused by Borrelia infection (Lyme's disease), diphtheria, drugs, or toxin exposure • Nonhereditary • Without prominent sphincter disturbance • Not meeting the criteria for multifocal motor neuropathy, IgM with high titer anti-MAG antibodies, POEMS syndrome, osteosclerotic myeloma, diabetic or nondiabetic lumbosacral radiculoplexus neuropathy, lymphoma, and amyloidosis	
Electro-physiological criteria	*Definite*: Includes at least one of the following: • Prolonged motor distal latency ≥50% upper limit of normal (ULN) in 2 nerves (not including median nerve at wrist) • Reduced motor conduction velocity ≥30% below lower limit of normal (LLN) in 2 nerves • Prolonged F-wave latency ≥30% above ULN in 2 nerves (≥50% if amplitude of compound muscle action potential <80% below LLN) • Absent F-waves in 2 nerves if these nerves have CMAP ≥20% of LLN + ≥1 demyelinating parameter in ≥1 other nerve • Partial motor conduction block ≥50% amplitude reduction of proximal CMAP relative to distal (provided distal CMAP ≥ 20% of LLN) in 2 nerves, or in 1 nerve + ≥1 demyelinating parameter in ≥1 other nerve • Abnormal temporal dispersion (>30% duration increases between the proximal and distal CMAP) in ≥2 nerves • Distal CMAP duration increases in ≥1 nerve (median ≥ 6.6 ms; ulnar ≥ 6.7 ms; peroneal ≥ 7.6 ms; tibial ≥ 8.8 ms) + ≥1 demyelinating parameter in ≥1 other nerve *Probable*: ≥30% amplitude reduction of proximal CMAP relative to distal (provided distal CMAP ≥ 20% of LLN) in 2 nerves (except posterior tibial nerve), or in 1 nerve + ≥1 demyelinating parameter in ≥1 other nerve *Possible*: Any of the electrophysiologic criteria for definite CIDP, but in 1 nerve only	

Continued

Continued

Clinical criteria	Typical	Atypical
Supportive tests	• Elevated CSF protein with leukocyte count < 10 cells/mm^3 • MRI gadolinium enhancement and/or hypertrophy of cauda equina, lumbosacral or cervical nerve roots, or the brachial or lumbosacral plexuses • Abnormal sensory nerve conduction study in at least 1 nerve ○ Normal sural with abnormal median or radial sensory nerve action potentials (SNAP) (except median nerve at wrist) ○ Sensory conduction velocity <80% of LLN or <70% if SNAP <80% of LLN ○ Delayed somatosensory evoked potentials without central nervous system involvement • Evidence of demyelination or remyelination by nerve biopsy with electron microscopy or teased fiber analysis	

(CIDP: chronic inflammatory demyelinating polyneuropathy; CMAP: compound muscle action potential; CSF: cerebrospinal fluid; DADS: distal acquired demyelinating symmetric; EFNS/PNS: European Federation of Neurological Societies/Peripheral Nerve Society; IgM: immunoglobulin M; MADSAM: multifocal acquired demyelinating sensory and motor neuropathy; MAG: myelin-associated glycoprotein; POEMS: polyneuropathy, organomegaly, endocrinopathy, M protein, skin changes)

Q24. What are the common clues toward a diagnosis of Charcot–Marie–Tooth disease?

Ans.

- Very slowly progressive, distal symptoms
- Usually not majorly disabling
- Lower limb predominant involvement
- Wasting > Weakness
- Involvement of the calf and foot muscles leading to pes cavus and hammer toes; champagne bottle appearance of legs
- Family history of similar illness[22]

Q25. What is POEMS syndrome?

Ans. *POEMS syndrome* is a rare paraneoplastic neuropathy secondary to an underlying plasma cell dyscrasia. The diagnosis is confirmed when both mandatory, one of the three major and one of the six minor criteria are fulfilled **(Table 13)**.[23]

Q26. How do you diagnose amyotrophic lateral sclerosis?

Ans. Clinical examination is the most important for diagnosing amyotrophic lateral sclerosis (ALS) and determining simultaneous upper motor neuron (UMN) and lower motor neuron (LMN) involvement. The level of diagnostic certainty is thereafter based on the El Escorial criteria into possible, probable,

TABLE 13: POEMS syndrome.	
Mandatory criteria	• Polyneuropathy (typically demyelinating) • Monoclonal plasma cell-proliferative disorder (almost always lambda)
Major criteria	• Castleman disease • Sclerotic bone lesions • VEGF elevation
Minor criteria	• Organomegaly (splenomegaly, hepatomegaly, or lymphadenopathy) • Extravascular volume overload (edema, pleural effusion, and ascites) • Endocrinopathy (adrenal, thyroid, gonadal, pituitary, parathyroid, and pancreatic) • Skin changes (hyperpigmentation, hypertrichosis, plethora, acrocyanosis, flushing, and white nails) • Papilledema • Thrombocytosis/polycythemia

(POEMS: polyneuropathy, organomegaly, endocrinopathy, M protein, skin changes; VEGF: vascular endothelial growth factor)

and definite depending on the number of segments with UMN + LMN involvement (bulbar, cervical, thoracic, and lumbosacral). Nerve conduction velocity and electromyography (NCV/EMG) are important for diagnosis with findings of positive sharp waves or fibrillation potentials on EMG considered equivalent to LMN involvement (in affected or unaffected muscles).

Recently, the Awaji criteria incorporated the presence of fasciculations (clinical/electrophysiological) as suggestive of LMN involvement.

All other potential etiologies for these findings should be ruled out. The false positive rate of diagnosis is between 8 and 10%.[24]

Q27. What are the treatment options available for amyotrophic lateral sclerosis at present?

Ans. *Riluzole* (dose: 50 mg BD; oral) is the only drug that has demonstrated the ability to increase survival in ALS patients, albeit by a few months.

Edaravone is a neuroprotectant, which acts as a free radical scavenger. It is transfused intravenously in a dose of 60 mg daily for 2 weeks followed by a 2-week drug-free period. Subsequent cycles consist of the same dose prescribed for 10–14 days, followed by a 2-week washout period. Although approved by the Food and Drug Administration (FDA), recent trials have shown treatment with edaravone to be well tolerated but having no significant effect in slowing disease progression, respiratory dysfunction or corticospinal tract degeneration on neuroimaging.

A recent phase 2 trial of perampanel in ALS failed to show any improvement in survival or decrease in disability. It rather showed an increase risk of adverse effects and more rapid decline in Revised Amyotrophic Lateral

Sclerosis Functional Rating Scale (ALSFRS-R) scores in the perampanel group.

Similarly, phase 2 and 3 trials of rapamycin, levosimendan, and reldesemtiv showed good safety profiles but could not demonstrate efficacy.

Tofersen in an FDA-approved treatment for *SOD1* mutation associated ALS. It is an antisense oligonucleotide targeting *SOD1* mutations, which showed mild clinical efficacy with significant effect on disease biomarkers like SOD1 and neurofilaments. Open-label extension of its pivotal trial is presently ongoing.

High-calorie therapy was a nonpharmacological therapy tried in ALS, which showed weight gain and body mass index (BMI) but no improvement in muscle strength or ALSFRS-R decline.[24]

Q28. What are the genetic aspects of juvenile-onset amyotrophic lateral sclerosis?

Ans. Juvenile onset is a neurodegenerative disorder with UMN and LMN dysfunction (ALS), with disease onset before 25 years of age. 40% of juvenile ALS cases have a genetic contribution. The most commonly involved genes and their characteristic features are mentioned **(Table 14)**.[25]

Q29. What are the differential diagnosis of amyotrophic lateral sclerosis?

Ans. Table 15 shows the differential diagnosis of ALS.[26]

TABLE 14: The genetic aspects of juvenile-onset ALS.

Gene mutation	*FUS*	*SETX*	*ALS2*	*SOD1*	*SPTLC1*
Inheritance	De novo	AD	AR	De novo	AR
Age of onset	Early third decade	Second decade	Early first decade	Late second decade	second to third decade
Initial symptom	Bulbar	Distal leg	Bulbar	Asymmetric, LMN	Bulbar and distal
Progression	Rapid	Slow	Slow	Rapid	Slow
Other characteristics	Myoclonus, tremor	Cerebellar findings	Scoliosis, anarthria	None	None
Cognitive impairment	Occasional	None	Pseudobulbar affect	None	None
MRI findings	Frontal cortical atrophy, pyramidal tract signal	None	Mild cortical + spinal cord atrophy	None	None

(AD: autosomal dominant; ALS: amyotrophic lateral sclerosis; AR: autosomal recessive; LMN: lower motor neuron)

TABLE 15: Differential diagnosis of ALS.

Predominant signs	Mimic disorder	Diagnostic clues
LMN	Benign fasciculations	No weakness
	MMNCB	Weakness > wasting, predilection for finger extensors, slowly progressive
	Neuralgic amyotrophy	Severe pain at onset; plateau and recovery
	Kennedy's disease	Very slow progression, sensory symptoms, gynecomastia, chin fasciculations
	Motor CIDP	Symmetrical, fluctuating, mild sensory involvement
	Inclusion body myositis	Slowly progressive; predilection for quadriceps and medial forearms
UMN	Hereditary spastic paraparesis	Younger onset, slow progression, family history, and mild or no upper limb involvement
	PPMS	Slowly progressive, MRI evidence of demyelination, and oligoclonal bands in CSF
UMN + LMN	Cervical myeloradiculopathy	Neck pain and bladder involvement

(CIDP: chronic inflammatory demyelinating polyneuropathy; CSF: cerebrospinal fluid; LMN: lower motor neuron; MMNCB: multifocal motor neuropathy with conduction block; PPMS: primary progressive multiple sclerosis; UMN: upper motor neuron)

TABLE 16: Different types of motor neuron diseases (MNDs).

MND type	Features
Amyotrophic lateral sclerosis	UMN + LMN features
Progressive bulbar palsy	LMN brainstem involvement
Primary lateral sclerosis	Pure UMN involvement
Progressive muscular atrophy	Pure LMN involvement

(LMN: lower motor neuron; UMN: upper motor neuron)

Q30. What are different types of motor neuron diseases?

Ans. Table 16 shows different types of motor neuron diseases.[26]

Q31. What is Kennedy's disease? How does it differ from classical motor neuron disease?

Ans. *Kennedy's disease* is a spinal and bulbar muscular atrophy (SBMA). It is a rare, X-linked LMN disease caused by an expanded trinucleotide repeat (CAG > 37) on the androgen receptor gene. This accumulation leads to toxicity affecting both motor neurons and muscles and is characterized by progressive quadriparesis, dysphagia, and dysarthria.[27]

It differs from motor neuron disease in the following aspects:

- Pure LMN syndrome
- Perioral myokymia—quivering chin
- Sensory symptoms—numbness and tingling
- Non-neurological manifestations—gynecomastia, testicular atrophy, infertility, and erectile dysfunction
- Laboratory findings—elevated creatine phosphokinase (CPK), diabetes, dyslipidemia, and nonalcohol fatty liver disease
- Nerve conduction study (NCS)—decreased sensory nerve action potentials

Q32. What is Hirayama disease? How does it differ from classical motor neuron disease?

Ans. Hirayama disease manifests as an insidious onset and gradually progressive weakness of the small muscles of hand and distal forearm muscles with sparing of the brachioradialis and musculature of the arm. It usually affects males in their late teenage years or early 20s and results from the forward displacement of the posterior dura, resulting in cervical compression on forward flexion of the neck. The disease usually plateaus after progressing for 2–5 years.[28]

Hirayama disease differs from ALS in the ways mentioned in **Table 17**.

TABLE 17: Difference between Hirayama disease and ALS.

	Hirayama disease	ALS
Onset	Late teens—early 20s	Fifth to sixth decade
Gender	Predominantly male	No gender-specific predisposition
Progression	2–5 years followed by plateau	Relentlessly progressive
Prognosis	• Good • No effect on life expectancy	• Poor • Usually leads to mortality 2–5 years after symptom onset
Etiology	Forward displacement of the posterior dura, resulting in cervical compression on forward flexion of the neck	No exact reason known
Neurological findings	• Pure LMN syndrome • Mostly unilateral and monomelic	• UMN + LMN findings • Bilateral and asymmetrical involvement
Treatment	• Cervical collar • Surgery	• Riluzole • Edaravone • Largely ineffective
Genetic forms	Not described	Familial ALS is known

(ALS: amyotrophic lateral sclerosis; LMN: lower motor neuron; UMN: upper motor neuron)

TABLE 18: Medical treatments for spinal muscular atrophy.

	Nusinersen	Onasemnogene Abeparvovec	Risdiplam
Drug type	Antisense oligonucleotide	Adeno-associated viral vector	Small molecule
Mechanism of action	Modification of SMN2 pre-mRNA splicing	*SMN* gene transfer	Modification of SMN2 pre-mRNA splicing
Route of administration	Intrathecal	Intravenous	Oral
Patient age	All	<2 years	>2 months
Clinical trials	• ENDEAR • CHERISH • NURTURE	• START • SPRINT	• FIREFISH • SUNFISH • RAINBOWFISH

Q33. What are the medical treatments for spinal muscular atrophy?

Ans. Spinal muscular atrophy (SMA) is an autosomal recessively inherited LMN disease, which leads to progressive proximal muscle weakness. The FDA-approved treatments for SMA are shown in **Table 18**.[29]

Q34. What are clinical features and diagnostics of hypokalemic periodic paralysis?

Ans. *Consensus diagnostic criteria for diagnosing hypokalemic periodic paralysis include*:

- ≥2 attacks of muscle weakness associated with serum potassium < 3.5 mEq/L

  or
- 1 attack of muscle weakness in the patient and 1 attack of muscle weakness in 1 relative with serum potassium < 3.5 mEq/L

  or
- ≥3 of the following:
  - Onset in the first or second decade
  - Duration of attack >2 hours
  - Presence of triggers (prior carbohydrate rich meal, symptom onset following rest after an exercise)
  - Improvement in symptoms after potassium intake
  - Family history of the condition or genetically confirmed skeletal calcium or sodium channel mutation
  - Positive long exercise test

  and
- Exclusion of other causes of hypokalemia such as drugs, toxins, renal, adrenal, and thyroid dysfunction
- Absence of myotonia[30]

TABLE 19: Management of a patient with diabetic neuropathy.

Oral pharmacological agents	Anticonvulsants	• Pregabalin • Gabapentin
	Tricyclic antidepressants	• Nortriptyline • Amitriptyline • Desipramine • Imipramine
	Serotonin–norepinephrine reuptake inhibitors	• Desvenlafaxine • Duloxetine • Venlafaxine
	Tramadol	
	Tapentadol	
	Opioid agonists	• Oxycodone • Methadone
Topical agents	Capsaicin	
	Lidocaine	
	Clonidine gel	
	Isosorbide dinitrate spray	

Q35. How to manage a patient with diabetic neuropathy?

Ans. Table 19 shows the management of a patient with diabetic neuropathy.[31]

REFERENCES

1. Khadilkar SV, Yadav RS, Patel BA (Eds). Neuromuscular Disorders: A Comprehensive Review with Illustrative Cases. Mumbai: Springer; 2018.
2. Lewis SL. CONTINUUM: Lifelong learning in neurology. Muscle and Neuromuscular Junction Disorders. 2022;28(6):1576-9.
3. Khadilkar SV, Chaudhari CR, Patil TR, Desai ND, Jagiasi KA, Bhutada AG. Once myasthenic, always myasthenic? observations on the behavior and prognosis of myasthenia gravis in a cohort of 100 patients. Neurol India. 2014;62(5):492-7.
4. Nadkarni JJ, Dastur RS, Viswanathan V, Gaitonde PS, Khadilkar SV. Duchenne and Becker muscular dystrophies: An Indian update on genetics and rehabilitation. Neurol India. 2008;56(3):248-53.
5. Khadilkar SV, Faldu HD, Patil SB, Singh R. Limb-girdle muscular dystrophies in India: A review. Ann Indian Acad Neurol. 2017;20:87-95.
6. Khadilkar SV. Muscular dystrophy: The long road ahead. Neurol India. 2017;65:968.
7. Khadilkar SV, Patil SG, Amin SN. Study of idiopathic inflammatory myopathies with special reference to borderland between idiopathic inflammatory myopathies and muscular dystrophy. Neurol India. 2008;56(3):356-62.
8. Khadilkar SV, Patel BA, Lalkaka JA. Making sense of the clinical spectrum of limb girdle muscular dystrophies. Pract Neurol. 2018;18(3):201-10.
9. Khadilkar SV, Soni GS (Eds). Neurology Simplified, 3rd edition. Mumbai: The National Book Depot; 2020.
10. Stevens D, Milani-Nejad S, Mozaffar T. Pompe Disease: a Clinical, Diagnostic, and Therapeutic Overview. Curr Treat Options Neurol. 2022;24(11):573-88.

11. Bouchard C, Tremblay JP. Limb–Girdle Muscular Dystrophies Classification and Therapies. J Clin Med. 2023;12:4769.
12. Mishra AK, Varma A. Myasthenia Gravis: A Systematic Review. Cureus. 2023;15(12):e50017.
13. Dresser L, Wlodarski R, Rezania K, Soliven B. Myasthenia Gravis: Epidemiology, Pathophysiology and Clinical Manifestations. J Clin Med. 2021;10:2235.
14. Iorio R. Myasthenia gravis: the changing treatment landscape in the era of molecular therapies. Nat Rev Neurol. 2024;20:84-98.
15. Thomas PK, Ochoa J. Symptomatology and differential diagnosis of peripheral neuropathy. In: Dyck PJ, Thomas PK (Eds). Peripheral Neuropathy. Philadelphia: Saunders; 1993. pp. 749-74.
16. Kleyweg RP, van der Meche FGA, Schmitz PIM. Interobserver agreement in the assessment of muscle strength and functional abilities in Guillain-Barré syndrome. Muscle Nerve. 1991;14(11):1103-9.
17. Walgaard C, Lingsma HF, Ruts L, Drenthen J, van Koningsveld R, Garssen MJ, et al. Prediction of respiratory insufficiency in Guillain-Barré syndrome. Ann Neurol. 2010;67:781-7.
18. Asbury AK, Cornblath DR. Assessment of current diagnostic criteria for Guillain-Barré syndrome. Ann Neurol. 1990;27:S21-S24.
19. Leonhard SE, Mandarakas MR, Gondim FAA, Bateman K, Ferreira MLB, Cornblath DR, et al. Diagnosis and management of Guillain-Barré syndrome in ten steps. Nat Rev Neurol. 2019;15:671-83.
20. Jones MR, Urits I, Wolf J, Corrigan D, Colburn L, Peterson E, et al. Drug induced peripheral neuropathy: A narrative review. Curr Clin Pharmacol. 2020;15:38-48.
21. van den Bergh PYK, van Doorn PA, Hadden RDM, Avau B, Vankrunkelsven P, Allen JA, et al. European Academy of Neurology/Peripheral Nerve Society guideline on diagnosis and treatment of chronic inflammatory demyelinating polyradiculoneuropathy: Report of a joint Task Force-Second revision. J Peripher Nerv Syst. 2021;26(3):242-68.
22. Nagappa M, Sharma S, Taly AB. (2024). Charcot-Marie-Tooth Disease. StatPearls. Treasure Island (FL): StatPearls Publishing. [online] Available from https://www.ncbi.nlm.nih.gov/books/NBK562163/ [Last accessed January, 2025].
23. Dispenzieri A. POEMS syndrome: 2021 update on diagnosis, risk-stratification, and management. Am J Hematol. 2019;94:812-27.
24. Riva N, Domi T, Pozzi L, Lunetta C, Schito P, Spinelli EG, et al. Update on recent advances in amyotrophic lateral sclerosis. J Neurol. 2024;271:4693-723.
25. Lehky T, Grunseich C. Juvenile amyotrophic lateral sclerosis: a review. Genes. 2021;12:1935.
26. Turner MR, Talbot K. Mimics and chameleons in motor neuron disease. Pract Neurol. 2013;13:153-64.
27. Breza M, Koutsis G. Kennedy's Disease (spinal and bulbar muscular atrophy): a clinically oriented review of a rare disease. J Neurol. 2019;266(3):565-73.
28. Gomathy SB, Priyanka Y, Garg A, Macken WL, Agarwal A, Ahmed T, et al. Phenotypic, electrophysiologic, and imaging spectrum of Hirayama disease from Northern India. Ann Ind Acad Neurol. 2024;27(5):524-9.
29. Nishio H, Niba ETE, Saito T, Okamoto K, Takeshima Y, Awano H. Spinal muscular atrophy: the past, present, and future of diagnosis and treatment. Int J Mol Sci. 2023;24(15):11939.
30. Statland JM, Fontaine B, Hanna MG, Johnson NE, Kissel JT, Sansone VA, et al. Review of the Diagnosis and Treatment of Periodic Paralysis. Muscle Nerve. 2018;57(4):522-30.
31. Gandhi M, Fargo E, Prasad-Reddy L, Mahoney KM, Isaacs D. Diabetes: how to manage diabetic peripheral neuropathy. Drugs Context. 2022;11:2021-10-2.

SECTION 3

Functional Neurology

Section Editors: Sudhir Kothari, Hrishikesh Kumar

Associate Editors: Soaham Desai, Jacky Ganguly

OVERVIEW

Functional neurological disorders (FNDs) are an increasingly recognized area in neurology and psychiatry. Once misunderstood and stigmatized, FND is now seen as a well-defined condition, supported by modern neuroscience and imaging techniques. It has become the second most common reason for outpatient neurology visits, making it a vital topic for clinical practice. FND highlights the connection between neurology and psychiatry, offering insights into how biological, psychological, and social factors influence symptoms.

To help readers better understand and approach this important topic, we have carefully curated a set of key questions and answers. These address the definition of FND, mechanisms, diagnostic methods, history-taking, examination techniques, treatment strategies, and subtypes. Our aim is to introduce readers to the core concepts of FND and provide practical guidance for managing patients with these conditions.

We hope this resource not only clarifies the basics but also sparks further interest in this rapidly evolving field. For those who wish to explore the subject in more depth, we have given a list of some additional reading material at the end of the document.

- **What are functional neurological disorders (FNDs)?**
  Functional neurological disorders are genuine neurological conditions caused by disrupted brain networks and abnormal signal processing, leading to motor, sensory, and cognitive symptoms without structural abnormalities. Symptoms are real, involuntary, and diagnosed based on positive clinical signs.
  For details, see Q1.

- **Are FNDs genuine disorders?**
  Functional neurological disorders have been shown to be genuine disorders caused by disruptions in brain connectivity and processing networks. Neuroimaging studies reveal altered patterns of activation that

validate their biological basis. Symptoms are involuntary, not fabricated, and result from dysfunction rather than damage.
For legitimacy and neuroimaging evidence, see Q2.

- **Why use the term "FND"?**
The term "FND" replaces outdated labels like "hysteria" and "conversion disorder" that carried stigma and implied psychological causation. Modern terminology emphasizes the biological basis of symptoms, promoting acceptance, reducing stigma, and encouraging patient engagement.
For terminology and historical context, refer to Q3.
- **Diagnosis: Rule-in approach and positive signs**
The rule-in approach uses positive signs during examination, such as Hoover's sign and tremor entrainment, to confirm FND. This contrasts with older methods that relied on exclusion, reducing stigma and enabling earlier intervention.
For diagnostic criteria and examples of positive signs, see Q4.
- **Variability, distractibility, and inconsistency in diagnosis**
Variability, distractibility, and inconsistency are key features of FND. Symptoms may change over time, improve with distraction, and lack anatomical consistency. These features help distinguish FND from organic disorders and demonstrate reversibility.
For more details, see Q5.
- **Role of stressors in diagnosis**
Stressors may be present in some cases of FND, but their absence does not exclude the diagnosis. Diagnosis relies on positive clinical signs rather than psychological histories, as FND can occur without identifiable stress or trauma.
For further explanation, see Q6.
- **How to broach the topic of stress?**
Discussing stress in FND requires sensitivity and nonstigmatizing language. Focus should be on building trust, explaining the link between stress and symptoms, and normalizing stress as a contributing factor rather than the sole cause.
For communication strategies, see Q7.
- **FND with preexisting neurological disorders**
Functional neurological disorder can coexist with preexisting neurological conditions such as epilepsy, multiple sclerosis, or stroke. Identifying functional symptoms alongside organic disorders ensures accurate diagnosis and prevents mismanagement.
For more details, see Q8.
- **Pitfalls in diagnosis and how to avoid them**
Diagnostic pitfalls include misattributing symptoms to stress, over-relying on exclusion, and failing to identify positive signs. Careful evaluation and use of positive signs reduce errors and prevent misdiagnosis.
For detailed strategies, see Q9.

- **Risks of missing diagnosis**
  Missed diagnoses may lead to unnecessary investigations, delayed treatment, and psychological distress. Recognizing positive signs early and ensuring multidisciplinary care helps mitigate these risks.
  For further details, see Q10.
- **Risks of overdiagnosis in FND**
  Overdiagnosis can result in missed organic diagnoses, inappropriate treatments, psychological harm, and delayed recovery. Careful evaluations and a rule-in approach are essential to prevent these risks.
  For strategies to avoid overdiagnosis, see Q11.
- **Neurological assessment and communication as therapy**
  Neurological assessments provide both diagnostic and therapeutic opportunities. Demonstrating reversibility, validating symptoms, and communicating clearly foster trust and encourage recovery.
  For examples and approaches, see Q12.
- **Practical approach to management**
  Managing FND involves the biopsychosocial model, focusing on education, symptom relief, and rehabilitation. Medications support psychiatric comorbidities, while referrals and team-building improve care access.
  For practical management strategies, see Q13.
- **Roles of the neurologist and psychiatrist**
  Neurologists remain central to diagnosis, patient education, and ongoing care, while psychiatrists address psychological aspects. Multidisciplinary collaboration ensures holistic management.
  For detailed roles, see Q14.
- **Case example: Sudden limb weakness**
  Sudden limb weakness requires distinguishing functional causes from structural lesions. Positive signs like Hoover's test and distractibility help differentiate FND from organic conditions.
  For assessment strategies, see Q15.
- **Functional seizures**
  Functional seizures mimic epileptic seizures but lack abnormal electrical activity on electroencephalogram (EEG). Diagnosis relies on clinical features, video EEG, and history, with management focusing on psychological therapy and education.
  For detailed evaluation and management, see Q16.
- **Functional sensory symptoms**
  Functional sensory symptoms include non-anatomical patterns like glove-and-stocking distribution, inconsistent findings, and preserved reflexes. Diagnosis is based on positive signs and inconsistency across examinations.
  For further details, see Q17.

- **Functional coma**
  Functional coma presents with preserved reflexes, resistance to eye opening, and no structural or metabolic cause. Diagnosis depends on ruling out organic causes and identifying inconsistency in responses.
  For diagnostic and management approaches, see Q18.
- **Functional gait disorder**
  Functional gait disorders feature inconsistent patterns, exaggerated effort, and variability. Diagnosis relies on recognizing incongruent movements and ensuring rehabilitation through physiotherapy and education.
  For evaluation strategies, see Q19.
- **Persistent postural perceptual dizziness (PPPD)**
  This is characterized by chronic dizziness and hypersensitivity to motion. It often follows vestibular insults or stress and is managed through vestibular rehabilitation, cognitive behavioral therapy (CBT), and pharmacotherapy.
  For diagnostic criteria and management, see Q20.
- **Functional movement disorders**
  Functional movement disorders include tremors, dystonia, and gait abnormalities. Diagnosis relies on variability, distractibility, and inconsistency, with treatment focusing on physiotherapy, psychoeducation, and CBT.
  For diagnosis and management strategies, see Q21.
- **Functional tremors**
  Functional tremors often mimic organic tremors but show variability, distractibility, and entrainment. Diagnostic tests such as rhythm tasks and distraction techniques confirm the diagnosis.
  For detailed evaluation, see Q22.
- **Functional parkinsonism**
  Functional parkinsonism mimics idiopathic Parkinson's disease but differs in sudden onset, distractibility, and reversibility. Diagnosis relies on identifying inconsistencies and ruling out organic causes.
  For evaluation and treatment approaches, see Q23.
- **Intermittent abnormal movements**
  Intermittent abnormal movements in FNDs differ from dystonia or chorea due to variability, atypical triggers, and suggestibility. Diagnosis requires identifying inconsistencies and emphasizing functional features.
  For further explanations, see Q24.
- **Sudden visual loss**
  Functional vision loss presents with nonanatomical patterns, preserved reflexes, and normal imaging. Diagnosis involves behavioral tests and neurophysiological evaluations to confirm intact visual processing.
  For diagnostic approaches and treatments, see Question 25.

- **Functional eye movements**
  Functional eye movement abnormalities include convergence spasm and oculomotor disturbances. Diagnosis is based on inconsistencies and variability, with treatments focusing on education and targeted rehabilitation.
  For diagnostic and management approaches, see Q26.
- **Functional cognitive symptoms and memory loss**
  Functional cognitive symptoms include memory lapses, brain fog, and concentration difficulties. Diagnosis depends on inconsistencies and preserved functioning under distraction, while treatment emphasizes psychoeducation and CBT.
  For further details, see Q27.
- **Functional voice and speech disorders**
  Functional voice and speech disorders present as sudden loss of voice, stuttering, or changes in articulation. Diagnosis relies on variability and reversibility, and treatment involves speech therapy and relaxation techniques.
  For evaluation and management, see Q28.
- **Functional urinary problems**
  Functional urinary symptoms include retention, urgency, and frequency without identifiable structural abnormalities. Diagnosis depends on inconsistency, and treatment focuses on pelvic physiotherapy and behavioral therapy.
  For further explanations, see Q29.
- **FND in children**
  FND in children often presents with motor and sensory symptoms and may coexist with anxiety or stress. Diagnosis follows the same principles as in adults, and treatment prioritizes reassurance, physiotherapy, and counseling.
  For detailed approaches, see Q30.
- **Clinical scenarios**
  Real-life clinical scenarios illustrate common FND presentations, diagnostic approaches, and management strategies. These examples help demonstrate practical application of FND principles.
  For specific case studies, see Q31.

CONCLUSION

Functional neurological disorder is a legitimate neurological disorder with distinct diagnostic criteria and effective treatments. This overview highlights key principles in diagnosis, communication, and management. For detailed exploration, refer to the corresponding questions.

Q1. What are functional neurological disorders, and how do they differ from other neurological conditions?

Ans. *Functional neurological disorders (FNDs)* are legitimate neurological conditions, where patients exhibit symptoms that are not attributable to structural, electrophysiological, or conventional pathological abnormalities. FNDs involve genuine disruptions in brain function, specifically in networks responsible for motor, sensory, and cognitive control.

Key characteristics of FNDs:

- *Pathophysiological basis*:
    - FNDs are associated with dysfunction in brain networks and abnormal neural signal processing.
    - Advanced neuroimaging reveals altered connectivity and measurable brain activity changes.
    - Symptoms are not under voluntary control and are not intentionally produced.
- *Clinical manifestations*:
    - *Motor symptoms*: Weakness, tremor, dystonia, gait disturbances
    - *Sensory symptoms*: Numbness, altered sensation, visual disturbances
    - *Seizure-like episodes*: Psychogenic nonepileptic seizures (PNES) that mimic epilepsy but lack electrophysiological correlates
    - *Cognitive symptoms*: Difficulty concentrating, memory disturbances
    - Symptoms are typically inconsistent or incongruent with known neurological disease patterns.
- *Diagnostic characteristics*:
    - *Positive signs*: Examples include Hoover's sign for functional weakness, distractibility of tremor, or inconsistency in symptoms.
    - *Normal investigations*: Structural imaging and standard neurological tests are unremarkable.
    - Symptoms often do not fit recognized neurological disease mechanisms.

Pathogenesis:

The etiology of FNDs involves complex interactions of:

- *Neurobiological mechanisms*: Abnormal brain connectivity and signal processing
- *Psychological factors*: Stress, trauma, or emotional conflicts
- *Predictive processing disruptions*: Brain's failure to integrate sensory input and motor output appropriately

CONCLUSION

Modern neuroscience confirms FNDs as genuine neurological conditions requiring understanding and empathy. Management emphasizes rehabilitation, neurological retraining, and psychological support, often delivered through multidisciplinary teams. These approaches target both brain and behavior, fostering symptom improvement and recovery.

Q2. Are functional disorders less genuine than organic ones, and how are they different from malingering?

Ans. Modern research in neuroscience now rejects old views that separate "organic" and "functional" disorders, showing that FNDs are genuine disorders caused by brain network dysfunction. While organic disorders involve structural or chemical abnormalities, FND reflects disrupted network activity and information processing. Both are valid neurological conditions requiring specific treatments.

How are functional disorders genuine?

Neuroimaging studies demonstrate distinct abnormalities in FND, proving they are rooted in brain dysfunction rather than being imagined or faked. Key findings include:

- Disrupted networks controlling movement, sensation, and self-awareness
- Changes in emotional-motor circuits, self-agency networks, and salience networks

Key networks involved:

- *Emotional motor circuits*: Overactive connections between emotional and motor areas result in abnormal movements and sensory responses. These circuits link emotional states to physical actions, explaining why stress can trigger or worsen symptoms.
- *Self-agency networks:* Dysfunction in the right temporoparietal junction impairs the sense of control over actions, leading to symptoms perceived as involuntary. This network processes the feeling of ownership and intention behind movements.
- *Salience networks*: Hyperactivity in regions like the anterior cingulate cortex and insula increases focus on symptoms and reduces attention regulation. These networks help prioritize important stimuli and regulate responses to perceived threats.

Key evidence from imaging:

- *Functional MRI (fMRI)*: It shows hyperactivation in emotional motor circuits and reduced connectivity in motor control networks.
- *Diffusion tensor imaging (DTI)*: Reveals weakened pathways between brain regions, explaining communication disruptions.
- *EEG and PET scans*: Highlight altered brain activity patterns, reinforcing the biological basis of symptoms.

How are they different from malingering?

Unlike malingering, where symptoms are intentionally faked for personal gain, FND symptoms occur unconsciously. Brain scans confirm real changes in activity during symptom episodes, distinguishing FND from deliberate simulation. Studies of functional tremors confirm movement patterns that cannot be voluntarily reproduced, validating that symptoms are involuntary.

Key differences from malingering:

- Functional neurological disorders symptoms are involuntary, arising from disrupted brain networks.
- Malingering involves conscious control and intent, without underlying neural abnormalities.
- Imaging studies provide objective evidence for FND, ruling out intentional deception.

Role of attention networks: Problems with attention may play a central role in FND. Imaging studies show:

- Overactive emotional motor circuits during symptom focus
- Poor suppression of the brain's default mode during tasks
- Weak links between attention and motor networks

This suggests symptoms result from disrupted attention-motor pathways, not deliberate actions.

CONCLUSION

Functional neurological disorder is as genuine as organic disorders, arising from measurable brain dysfunction rather than conscious fabrication. Neuroimaging evidence supports FND as a legitimate condition, distinct from malingering. This understanding promotes accurate diagnosis, reduces stigma, and guides effective treatment strategies.

Q3. Why use the term "FND" instead of older terms like "Hysteria" or "Conversion Disorder"?

Ans.

Historical limitations of older terms:

- *Hysteria*: Historically linked to outdated and sexist beliefs, associating symptoms with the uterus. This term fostered dismissive attitudes, particularly toward women, and contributed to stigma.
- *Conversion disorder*: It implies that physical symptoms result from psychological distress being "converted" into bodily manifestations. This perspective can invalidate the patient's experience, leading to feelings of dismissal and frustration.

Modern understanding of FND:

The term "Functional Neurological Disorders" reflects advances in understanding these conditions as genuine neurological disorders, caused by functional brain network disruptions rather than structural abnormalities. This terminology emphasizes the reality of the symptoms without implying that they are fabricated, imagined, or secondary to psychological issues.

Functional neurological disorders aligns with current research, framing the condition as a dysfunction in how the brain processes signals, rather than as a purely psychological issue. This approach reduces stigma, making patients more likely to accept the diagnosis and engage in treatment.

Benefits for patients and Physicians:

- *Patient-centered care*: The term "FND" avoids language that may alienate patients, fostering a therapeutic environment based on trust. It emphasizes the reality of their symptoms, promoting acceptance and collaboration in care.
- *Improved communication*: Using FND ensures clarity and neutrality in discussions with patients and colleagues, reducing miscommunication or misunderstandings.
- *Multidisciplinary management*: The term highlights the need for an integrated approach that combines neurological, psychological, and rehabilitative care for optimal outcomes.

CONCLUSION

Adopting the term "FND" reflects a shift toward patient-centered, stigma-free care. It enhances trust, reduces patient disengagement, and ensures treatment is grounded in modern scientific understanding. For physicians, it ensures clear communication and encourages a comprehensive approach to manage these complex disorders.

Q4. How does the new approach of rule-in a diagnosis of functional neurological disorders differ from the earlier rule-out approach? What is the meaning of positive signs?

Ans. The new rule-in approach is very different from the earlier rule-out approach to diagnosis of FND, and we now use positive signs to make the diagnosis, like we do with other neurological disorders.

Earlier rule-out approach:

- *Diagnostic method*: Required ruling out all other organic or structural neurological conditions before diagnosing FND.
- *Implications*: Positioned FND as a "diagnosis of exclusion," implying it was a condition diagnosed by default rather than by specific criteria.
- *Stigma*: Reinforced the perception that FND was not a "real" neurological condition but a psychological or fabricated disorder.
- *Challenges*: Often delayed diagnosis and treatment as extensive investigations were conducted to eliminate other possibilities.

New rule-in approach:

- *Diagnostic method*: It focuses on identifying positive signs that actively confirm the diagnosis of FND based on unique clinical features.
- *Implications*: It frames FND as a legitimate, independent condition with specific diagnostic criteria, no longer relying on exclusion of other disorders.
- *Stigma reduction*: It validates FND as a neurological disorder with identifiable pathophysiology, improving patient trust and acceptance.
- *Efficiency*: It promotes earlier diagnosis and initiation of management without unnecessary testing.

What are positive signs?

Positive signs are specific, reproducible clinical findings that confirm the presence of FND. These signs distinguish FND from other conditions and support the diagnosis directly.

Examples:

- *Motor symptoms*:
    - Inconsistent or incongruent motor weakness
    - Variable tremors (amplitude/frequency)
    - Give-way weakness or positive Hoover's sign
    - Movements that do not follow recognized neurological patterns
- *Sensory symptoms*:
    - Nonanatomical sensory loss
    - Sensory disturbances not corresponding to neuroanatomical pathways
- *Cognitive/psychological features*:
    - Disproportionate emotional responses
    - Variable cognitive/attentional performance
    - Dissociative phenomena

Key differences:

The rule-in approach emphasizes diagnosing FND through its unique clinical signs rather than as a diagnosis of exclusion. It reframes FND as a genuine disorder requiring specific management, addressing stigma, and improving outcomes.

Q5. What is the place of variability, distractibility, and inconsistency in the diagnosis of functional neurological disorder?

Ans. Variability, distractibility, and inconsistency are the hallmark features of FND that help distinguish it from organic neurological conditions.

- *Variability*:
    - *Definition*: Symptoms in FND often change in intensity, location, or nature over time or during examinations.
    - *Key insight*: While variability is important, *incongruency*—symptoms that defy known neuroanatomical or physiological explanations—is a stronger diagnostic marker.
    - *Example*: Functional tremors may shift in pattern or intensity, unlike the predictable variability of Parkinson's tremor, which remains congruent with PD's characteristics.
- *Distractibility*:
    - *Definition*: Symptoms reduce or disappear when the patient's attention is diverted from the affected function.
    - *Key insight*: Distractibility is rarely seen in organic disorders and strongly suggests FND.

  - *Example*: A patient with a functional gait disorder may walk normally while engaged in conversation or a cognitive task.
- *Inconsistency*:
  - *Definition*: Discrepancies between reported symptoms and objective findings or known neuroanatomical principles
  - *Key insight*: Inconsistency highlights the mismatch between subjective deficits and objective examination.
  - *Example*: Functional sensory loss may follow a nonanatomical distribution (e.g., glove-and-stocking pattern), unlike deficits caused by nerve or spinal cord pathology.

Clinical utility:
- *Positive diagnosis*: These features provide affirmative evidence for FND, avoiding reliance on exclusion.
- *Differentiation*: They distinguish FND from organic conditions, which typically show consistent and anatomically congruent findings.
- *Therapeutic relevance*: Demonstrating these features helps patients understand their condition and engage with treatment.
- *Avoiding misdiagnosis*: Recognizing these involuntary features prevents mislabeling FND as malingering or factitious disorder.

Limitations:
- These features may not be present in all FND cases (e.g., functional dystonia).
- Should always be used alongside other diagnostic findings.

CONCLUSION

Variability, distractibility, and inconsistency are essential for diagnosing FND. They validate FND as a genuine condition, facilitate early diagnosis, and guide appropriate management.

Q6. In diagnosing functional neurological disorder, how much importance is to be given to the presence or absence of an obvious stressor?

Ans. Functional neurological disorders are characterized by neurological symptoms such as sudden weakness, abnormal movements, sensory disturbances or gait abnormalities, which are inconsistent with structural or organic pathology. Diagnosis focuses on identifying positive clinical signs rather than getting biased by the presence of stressors.

Role of stressors in diagnosis:
Stressors, such as quarrels or traumatic events, can act as precipitants for functional symptoms. However, their presence is neither necessary nor sufficient for diagnosis. FND can occur with or without identifiable stressors, as reflected in the Diagnostic and Statistical Manual of Mental Disorders,

Fifth edition (DSM-5) criteria. Stress can also trigger organic conditions, such as cerebrovascular events or demyelination, making it unreliable as a standalone diagnostic marker. While understanding stressors may provide context, diagnosis should focus on clinical features rather than psychosocial history.

Caution with stressor-based diagnosis:
Clinicians must be cautious about overemphasizing or dismissing stressors when diagnosing FND. An immediate stressor can lead to prematurely labeling symptoms as functional, potentially missing an organic cause. Conversely, the absence of an identifiable stressor can lead to overlooking FND in favor of extensive investigations for organic pathology. Both scenarios can delay appropriate diagnosis and management, highlighting the need to prioritize positive clinical signs over psychosocial factors.

Dispelling the stress/trauma requirement:
Modern research has shown that FND can arise through altered predictive processing, or network dysfunction, independent of psychological stressors. The rates of trauma or stress are comparable to many organic neurological conditions, with up to 25–40% patients not reporting any identifiable stressful events before symptom onset. Some patients develop symptoms after purely physical triggers such as viral infections, minor injuries, or medical procedures.

La Belle indifference:
An apparent lack of concern about symptoms was earlier noted as a pointer to FND. However, it is neither sensitive nor specific. It is seen in only about 21% of FND cases and can also appear in organic conditions, such as frontal lobe damage from stroke or neurodegenerative diseases. Thus reliance on this sign for diagnosis is inadequate and can lead to misinterpretation.

Better approach to assessment:

- *Primary focus*: Begin with a thorough neurological examination, identify positive clinical signs, and establish diagnosis based on these findings. Build therapeutic rapport by explaining physical signs clearly.
- *Secondary considerations*: Address psychological factors only later after confirming diagnosis and after building rapport. Recognize stress/trauma as potential contributors rather than primary causes and consider them as maintaining rather than initiating factors.
- *Diagnostic communication*: Avoid attributing symptoms solely to stress. Explain the diagnosis using models emphasizing nervous system dysfunction while validating the reality and involuntary nature of the symptoms.

CONCLUSION

Stressors and apparent indifference may raise suspicion of FND but are neither necessary nor sufficient for diagnosis. Clinicians should guard against being misled by the presence or absence of stressors—

overdiagnosing FND in cases with a stressor and underdiagnosing it in those without one. Positive clinical signs remain the cornerstone for identifying FND. Dispelling the outdated notion that stress or trauma is a prerequisite for FND diagnosis facilitates early intervention and better therapeutic relationships.

Q7. How and when should we broach the topic of depression, anxiety, stress, or past trauma?

Ans. *Introduction*: Addressing psychological factors such as depression, anxiety, stress, or past trauma in patients with FND requires sensitivity, timing, and a structured approach. Psychological factors are not the sole cause of FND but can interact with biological and social influences, contributing to symptom maintenance or exacerbation. Discussions must be framed to avoid stigma and defensiveness, fostering trust and encouraging patient engagement. This section focuses on practical strategies, including sample questions, for addressing these issues during diagnosis and management.

When to address psychological factors?

- *During diagnosis*:
  - Initial phase: Focus on validating the patient's symptoms and ruling in the diagnosis using positive signs rather than exclusion-based methods.
  - Build trust before probing: Early discussions should avoid direct exploration of psychological history, which may create mistrust or defensiveness.
  - Introduce subtly after symptom validation: Once physical symptoms are acknowledged as real, psychological factors can be gently introduced as a part of a holistic framework.

Example questions:

- "You mentioned that your symptoms started quite suddenly. Were there any major changes or stressful events in your life around that time?"
- "Have you noticed whether your symptoms feel worse during times of stress or when you are feeling anxious?"
- "It is not uncommon for the body to react physically to stress. Can we explore whether stress might be playing any role in how you have been feeling?"
- *During management*:
  - Timing after trust is established: Revisit psychological factors once the diagnosis is accepted and rapport is built.
  - Link psychological factors to symptom fluctuations: Focus on patterns rather than causes to keep discussions practical and nonjudgmental.
  - Emphasize the mind-body connection: Explain that stress and emotions influence neurological functioning, similar to how anxiety causes palpitations.

Example questions:

- "Some of my other patients have found that stress or worry can sometimes worsen physical symptoms. Have you noticed anything like that?"
- "It is common for our bodies to hold tension or react physically to emotional stress. Do you think stress might be contributing to how your body is responding?"
- "Many people find that understanding emotional patterns helps them manage symptoms better. Would you be open to exploring this further?"

How to address psychological factors?

- *Normalize the role of emotions*: Frame emotions and stress as natural responses rather than as causes of the disorder.

Example explanation:

- "We know that the brain controls movements and sensations, but it also responds to stress in ways we do not always notice. This does not mean the symptoms are not real—it means we are understanding how the brain is reacting."
- *Avoid stigmatizing language*: Replace phrases like "psychological problem" or "in your head" with neutral terms such as "stress-related influences" or "brain network responses."
- *Use trauma-informed approaches*: Ask about trauma carefully, without implying causation or forcing disclosure.

Example questions:

- "I understand it can be difficult to talk about personal experiences, but sometimes past stress or trauma can affect how the brain processes information. Has anything like that ever been part of your experience?"
- "People who have been through stressful events often describe their bodies reacting in unexpected ways. Does that sound familiar to you?"
- *Collaborative inquiry*: Engage the patient as a partner in understanding their symptoms rather than imposing explanations.

Example questions:

- "You have described times when your symptoms get worse. Have you noticed whether these episodes happen during particularly stressful periods?"
- "We are learning that the brain and body are closely connected. Would you be open to exploring whether stress or emotions might be playing a role in what you are experiencing?"
- *Provide reassurance without dismissal*: Reassure patients that their symptoms are real and not imagined.

Example explanation:

- "What you are experiencing is very real, and many people with similar symptoms have found that understanding how stress affects the brain can be a helpful part of treatment. This does not mean the symptoms are in your head—it means we can work together to help your brain and body recover."

Key phrases to avoid:

- "It is all in your head."—Instead, say, "Your symptoms are real, and they are caused by changes in how the brain functions, not damage to the nerves."
- "You just need to relax."—Instead, say, "Stress management techniques can be one tool to help your brain regain balance."
- "You are imagining this."—Instead, say, "We know the brain can send signals that feel physical, even when scans look normal. This does not make it any less real."

CONCLUSION

Broaching the topic of psychological factors in FND requires timing, empathy, and nonjudgmental language. By validating symptoms early, establishing trust, and gradually introducing psychological factors as part of a holistic framework, clinicians can help patients feel supported rather than stigmatized. Using open-ended questions, trauma-informed approaches, and collaborative inquiry builds rapport and encourages patients to engage actively in their care.

Q8. Can you get FND in persons with preexisting neurological disorders? How to suspect in such patients?

Ans. Having a preexisting organic neurological disorder is itself a risk factor for developing FND, and so FND can coexist with established neurological conditions such as Parkinson's disease, epilepsy, and multiple sclerosis mimicking or amplifying preexisting organic symptoms, leading to potential misdiagnosis or delayed recognition.

How often do patients with neurological disorders develop superadded FND? Studies indicate that functional symptoms may coexist in 10–20% of cases. This overlap is often influenced by heightened awareness of symptoms, stress, or altered symptom perception, making diagnosis particularly challenging.

Organic disorders as a risk factor for FND: The presence of chronic illness may increase vulnerability due to heightened symptom monitoring, fear of progression, and psychological stress. These factors can amplify physical symptoms, leading to functional manifestations that coexist with the primary condition.

Key indicators to suspect FND in preexisting disorders:

- *Deviation from expected patterns*: Sudden onset or worsening of symptoms that do not fit the expected progression of the underlying disorder.
- *Inconsistencies*: Symptoms that fluctuate, improve with distraction, or lack anatomical or physiological correlation
- *Diagnostic tests*: Normal EEG during episodes resembling seizures or MRI findings inconsistent with reported symptoms in MS.

Condition-specific clues:

- *Parkinson's disease*: Tremors predominantly postural, disappearing with distraction, or sudden gait freezing without evidence of disease progression
- *Epilepsy*: Psychogenic nonepileptic seizures (PNES) presenting with preserved awareness, asynchronous movements, or lack of postictal confusion, confirmed by normal EEG during attacks
- *Multiple sclerosis*: Sensory symptoms like burning sensations or numbness that are inconsistent with imaging findings or anatomic pathways

Look for possible underlying organic disease even in definite FND:
Just because a patient has a definite diagnosis of FND does not exclude the presence of an underlying organic disorder. Both conditions can coexist, and careful evaluation is necessary to avoid overlooking treatable organic pathology.

It is important to recognize that functional symptoms may even mask an underlying organic disorder, which might only become apparent over time. For example, a patient initially presenting with definite functional seizures may have anticonvulsants discontinued based on a diagnosis of FND, only to later develop true epileptic seizures. This highlights the importance of ongoing clinical evaluation and follow-up to monitor symptom progression and response to treatment, ensuring that organic disorders are not missed.

CONCLUSION

Patients with preexisting neurological conditions can develop superadded FND, requiring careful evaluation to avoid misdiagnosis, and patients with definite FND can be subsequently found to have an underlying organic disease.

Diagnosis should rely on clinical patterns and key indicators, while maintaining awareness that functional symptoms do not rule out concurrent organic disease. Management should address both conditions through a multidisciplinary approach to ensure optimal care.

Q9. What are the pitfalls leading to misdiagnosis in functional neurological disorders (FND) and what strategies can one adopt to avoid them?

Ans. Functional neurological disorders present a diagnostic challenge due to their complex and overlapping symptomatology with organic and psychiatric conditions. While advances in understanding FND have led to improved diagnostic frameworks, errors in diagnosis—either overdiagnosis or missed/delayed diagnosis—remain significant concerns. Overdiagnosis often results from over-reliance on psychosocial stressors, incomplete examinations, or premature conclusions, while missed diagnoses arise from under-recognition of positive features specific to FND. This discussion highlights key pitfalls along with strategies to refine diagnostic accuracy, avoid overdiagnosis, and ensure timely identification of FND.

- *Pitfalls in history taking:*
  - *Overreliance on psychosocial stressors:* Assuming psychological stressors automatically indicate FND without ruling out organic causes.
    Example: Diagnosing FND in a patient with recent bereavement but overlooking early signs of multiple sclerosis.
  - *Incomplete history:* Failing to gather a detailed timeline of symptoms, associated features, or red flags (e.g., weight loss, fever, or progressive weakness).
    Example: Missing a history of nocturnal seizures in a patient presenting with episodic tremors.
  - *Patient bias:* Interpreting patient anxiety or distress as evidence of FND rather than a reaction to unexplained symptoms.
    Example: Labelling anxiety-driven hyperventilation as functional weakness without exploring organic causes.
  - *Lack of collateral history:* Not obtaining information from family or caregivers to corroborate symptoms or identify inconsistencies.
    Example: Overlooking reports of witnessed seizures inconsistent with psychogenic non-epileptic seizures (PNES).
- *Pitfalls in examination:*
  - *Overemphasis on positive signs of FND:* Relying solely on positive signs (e.g., Hoover's sign, tremor entrainment) without considering their specificity or limitations.
    Example: Diagnosing FND based on Hoover's sign alone without noticing mild spasticity indicative of early motor neuron disease.
  - *Incomplete neurological examination:* Missing subtle neurological signs (e.g., mild ataxia, reflex abnormalities) that could indicate an organic disorder.
    Example: Failing to detect brisk reflexes and Babinski sign in a patient later diagnosed with spinal cord compression.
  - *Misinterpretation of functional overlap:* Overlooking the coexistence of functional and organic symptoms (e.g., functional overlay in a patient with multiple sclerosis).
    Example: Misattributing gait disturbance in a patient with Parkinson's disease to FND alone.
- *Pitfalls in evaluation:*
  - *Premature diagnosis:* Diagnosing FND before completing a thorough workup to exclude organic conditions.
    Example: Attributing limb weakness to FND before conducting MRI to rule out stroke.
  - *Overreliance on normal investigations:* Assuming normal initial tests (e.g., MRI, EEG) rule out organic disease without considering their timing or sensitivity.

Example: Missing temporal lobe epilepsy due to a normal EEG during an interictal phase.

- *Inadequate follow-up:* Failing to reassess the diagnosis if symptoms evolve or do not respond to treatment.
  Example: Persisting with an FND diagnosis despite progressive muscle wasting suggesting motor neuron disease.

Situations prone to misdiagnosis of functional neurological disorder:

- *Subtle organic disorders:* Symptoms of early-stage multiple sclerosis, motor neuron disease, or epilepsy may initially mimic FND, leading to misdiagnosis.
- *Incomplete investigations:* Failing to perform advanced imaging or electrophysiological studies in cases with atypical symptoms.
- *Symptom fluctuation:* Organic conditions with fluctuating symptoms (e.g., demyelinating diseases) can be mistaken for functional symptoms.
- *Overlap with psychiatric disorders:* Coexisting psychiatric symptoms may mask underlying neurological diseases.
- *Communication barriers:* Misinterpretation of patient-reported symptoms due to language or cognitive difficulties.
- *Bias and assumptions:* Clinician bias toward psychological explanations in patients with prior psychiatric histories may overshadow physical findings.

Avoiding missed or delayed diagnosis of functional neurological disorder:

- *Recognize positive features early:* Train clinicians to identify hallmark features such as Hoover's sign, tremor entrainment, and inconsistency during examination.
- *Focus on rule-in diagnosis:* Emphasize identifying positive clinical signs rather than relying solely on exclusion.
- *Consider functional and organic overlap:* Evaluate the possibility of coexisting organic disorders to avoid premature conclusions.
- *Early specialist involvement:* Refer to neurologists or multidisciplinary teams when symptoms are complex or incongruent.
- *Use diagnostic tools effectively:* Employ imaging, electrophysiology, and neuropsychological testing to clarify unclear cases.
- *Patient education and engagement:* Explain the diagnosis clearly, ensuring patients understand their condition and remain actively involved in follow-up.
- *Monitor progress:* Track symptoms over time and reassess the diagnosis if treatment responses or symptoms deviate from expectations.

Key takeaway:

Balancing the diagnosis of FND requires a systematic, evidence-based approach that avoids both overdiagnosis and over-investigation. Physicians must prioritize thorough history-taking, careful examination, learning diagnosis by positive diagnostic criteria for FND and judicious use of investigations while maintaining open communication and regular follow-up with patients. Overdiagnosis of FND often arises in rushed evaluations, psychiatric overlays, and inexperienced assessments. Collaboration with multidisciplinary teams and ongoing education can further enhance diagnostic accuracy and patient care.

Q10. What is the risk or harm of missing a diagnosis of functional neurological disorder? What are the risk factors or pitfalls that can lead to missing diagnosis of functional neurological disorder?

Ans.

Risk and harm of missing diagnosis of FND:

Functional neurological disorders are common and treatable conditions, yet they are frequently misdiagnosed or overlooked in clinical practice. Failure to recognize FND can lead to significant physical, psychological, and social harm, along with unnecessary medical interventions and delays in the treatment.

Key risks of missed diagnosis:

- *Psychological and social harm*:
  - Misdiagnosing FND as other neurological conditions (e.g., epilepsy and stroke) may cause psychological distress, identity disruptions, and challenges with employment and relationships.
  - Patients may face social stigma and feelings of dismissal when diagnoses shift from organic to functional explanations.
- *Unnecessary medical treatments*:
  - Patients misdiagnosed with other conditions may undergo invasive procedures (e.g., surgeries or toxic drug therapies).
  - Functional seizures misdiagnosed as status epilepticus may lead to ICU admissions, complications such as infections, and respiratory issues.
- *Delay in appropriate treatment*:
  - Missed diagnosis delays therapies such as physiotherapy, psychotherapy, and rehabilitation, increasing the risk of chronicity and disability.
  - Late diagnosis erodes trust in healthcare providers, reducing patient engagement.
- *Diagnostic overshadowing and missed comorbidities*:
  - Attributing all symptoms to FND may result in overlooking coexisting psychiatric or neurological conditions.
  - Over-reliance on normal tests can lead to undertreatment of serious organic illnesses.
- *Emotional and financial burden*:
  - Patients face emotional stress and financial strain from repeated evaluations, missed work, and unnecessary tests.

Risk factors and pitfalls leading to missed diagnosis:

The diagnostic pitfalls leading to missed diagnoses of FND overlap significantly with those leading to *overdiagnosis*, as detailed in the earlier document. These include diagnostic bias, over-reliance on negative tests, symptom variability, lack of training, and rushed evaluations. However, additional risks unique to *missed diagnosis* include:

- *Fear of missing organic disorders*:
  - Clinicians may hesitate to diagnose FND without exhaustive testing, delaying recognition.
- *Inconsistent presentations*:
  - Fluctuating symptoms may lead to doubts about authenticity, increasing misinterpretation as malingering.
- *Emergency and acute settings*:
  - Pressure for rapid decisions in emergencies often leads to prioritizing life-threatening conditions, mislabeling FND as stroke or epilepsy.
- *Training deficiencies*:
  - Limited awareness and education about FND in medical curricula prevent clinicians from recognizing positive diagnostic signs like Hoover's sign or tremor entrainment.

Avoiding missed diagnosis:

- *Emphasize positive diagnostic features*: Reinforce training on identifying hallmark signs to make FND a rule-in diagnosis rather than one of exclusion.
- *Monitor progress and reassess*: Regularly evaluate symptoms and treatment responses to refine diagnosis.
- *Utilize multidisciplinary teams*: Collaborate with neurologists, psychiatrists, and physiotherapists for a comprehensive assessment.
- *Patient education*: Provide clear explanations to patients, minimizing stigma and improving engagement.

CONCLUSION

Missed diagnoses of FND result in profound harm due to psychological distress, unnecessary treatments, and delayed care. Addressing diagnostic challenges through education, multidisciplinary approaches, and patient-centered care can mitigate these risks. For a detailed discussion on pitfalls in *overdiagnosis* and strategies to avoid them, refer to the earlier document on diagnostic pitfalls in FND.

Q11. What are the risks, harm, and dangers of overdiagnosis in functional neurological disorders (FND)?

Ans.

Risks and harm of overdiagnosis in functional neurological disorders:

Overdiagnosis of functional neurological disorders (FND) occurs when the diagnosis is incorrectly applied to patients with underlying organic conditions or when made prematurely without comprehensive evaluation. This can lead to significant medical, psychological, and social consequences.

Key risks of overdiagnosis:

- *Missed organic diagnoses:*
  - Serious neurological or systemic conditions (e.g., epilepsy, stroke, multiple sclerosis, autoimmune diseases) may be overlooked. These could either be the actual diagnosis or comorbidities missed due to an exaggerated focus on FND.
  - Delayed or inappropriate treatment can result in disease progression and preventable complications.
    Example: A patient with functional seizures may have undiagnosed epilepsy, leading to uncontrolled seizures due to lack of antiseizure medicines.
- *Inappropriate treatment:*
  - Patients may receive psychological or rehabilitative therapies instead of necessary medical or surgical interventions.
  - This can exacerbate symptoms and delay effective management.
    Example: A patient with myasthenia gravis treated with psychotherapy instead of immunosuppressants may experience worsening muscle weakness.
- *Psychological harm:*
  - Misdiagnosis can lead to feelings of invalidation, stigma, and dismissal.
  - Patients may develop anxiety, depression, or mistrust in healthcare providers, potentially avoiding further care.
    Example: A patient misdiagnosed with FND may ignore progressive symptoms of multiple sclerosis, delaying critical treatment.
- *Increased healthcare costs:*
  - Unnecessary tests, therapies, and repeated evaluations escalate costs without addressing the underlying condition.
  - Financial burdens are imposed on both patients and healthcare systems.
    Example: Repeated psychotherapy sessions and psychiatric consultations for presumed FND without getting brain imaging may delay the diagnosis of a brain tumor, increasing treatment complexity and costs.
- *Medical harm:*
  - Unnecessary treatments, medications, or procedures can cause adverse effects, injuries, or disability.
    Example: A patient undergoing physiotherapy/chiropractic therapy/cupping therapy for functional weakness may develop ulcers, joint injuries, or chronic pain.
- *Erosion of trust in healthcare:*
  - Misdiagnosis can lead to loss of confidence in the healthcare system among patients and families.
  - Reduced compliance with medical advice and follow-ups may delay future diagnoses.
    Example: A patient with functional symptoms later diagnosed with Parkinson's disease may mistrust future treatments and avoid care.

- *Delayed recovery and poor outcomes:*
  - Prolonged misdiagnosis and inappropriate treatments delay effective interventions, leading to chronicity and worse prognoses.
    Example: A patient with autoimmune encephalitis misdiagnosed as FND may experience neurological deterioration before receiving immunotherapy.

Avoiding overdiagnosis:
Many diagnostic pitfalls overlap with those discussed in the earlier documents on *missed diagnoses* and *diagnostic pitfalls*. Strategies to avoid overdiagnosis include:

- *Thorough evaluations:* Complete history-taking, neurological examinations, and investigations before labeling symptoms as FND.
- *Rule-in approach:* Focus on positive diagnostic signs rather than exclusion.
- *Recognize overlaps:* Carefully assess for coexisting organic and functional features.
- *Consult multidisciplinary teams:* Collaborate with neurologists, psychiatrists, and rehabilitation specialists to ensure comprehensive evaluations.
- *Ongoing monitoring:* Reassess diagnosis if symptoms evolve or fail to respond to treatment.

CONCLUSION

Overdiagnosis of FND carries significant risks, including missed organic diagnoses, inappropriate treatments, psychological distress, financial strain, and medical harm. A thorough, evidence-based diagnostic approach is essential to minimize these dangers and ensure optimal patient care. For complementary strategies addressing *missed diagnoses* and *diagnostic pitfalls*, refer to earlier documents.

Q12. How can we use the neurological assessment and communication as treatment for functional neurological disorders (FND)?

Ans. Functional neurological disorders can be treated effectively starting with the neurological assessment itself. Beyond diagnosis, the assessment and communication process offer therapeutic opportunities by addressing fears, validating symptoms, and reinforcing the potential for recovery.

USING ASSESSMENT AS THERAPY

Building Trust and Validation

- Reassure patients that symptoms are *genuine* and *common*, reducing stigma and anxiety.
- Explain that FND is a disorder of *nervous system function,* not structural damage, which can be treated.

Positive Diagnostic Features

- Highlight *observable signs* such as Hoover's sign and tremor entrainment to reinforce a positive diagnosis rather than exclusion.
- Demonstrate reversibility of symptoms to boost confidence in recovery.

Example interaction:

- *Hoover's test*: "When you focus on your right leg, your left leg gets stronger. This shows that your nerves are intact, which is encouraging."
- *Tremor test*: "See how your tremor changes when you focus elsewhere? This tells us your nervous system can adapt."

Explaining Symptoms Mechanistically

- Use analogies, such as comparing FND to a *software glitch* rather than hardware damage, to help patients understand.

Example interaction:

- "Think of it as a software issue. The hardware is fine, but the messages are not being processed correctly. The good news is software problems can be fixed."

Therapeutic Demonstration During Examination

- Show patients how distraction improves movements, reinforcing symptom reversibility and treatment potential.

Example interaction:

- *Gait assessment*: "Let's walk while focusing on breathing or counting. Notice how that improves movement? Shifting focus can help retrain your brain."

Clarifying Diagnosis and Treatment Plan

- Clearly explain findings and emphasize that symptoms are *real and treatable.*
- Provide written resources, web links, and follow-up plans for reinforcement.

COMMUNICATING THE DIAGNOSIS OF FUNCTIONAL NEUROLOGICAL DISORDERS

Communicating the diagnosis is a pivotal step that determines patient perception, treatment adherence, and therapeutic alliance. Patients with FND often face frustration and dismissal, making clear and empathetic communication essential.

- *Validation and empathy:*
  - Acknowledge that symptoms are real, impactful, and debilitating.
  - Express understanding of prior frustrations with diagnostic uncertainty.

- *Positive framing of diagnosis:*
  - Emphasize that FND is a genuine, common, and treatable condition.
  - Avoid stigmatizing terms such as "psychogenic" or "imaginary." Frame FND as a *software problem* affecting brain processing, not a structural defect.
- *Empathetic analogies:*
  - Explain FND as a *signal processing disruption* that affects brain function but is reversible.
  - Highlight its prevalence (e.g., 16% of neurology outpatient visits) to normalize the diagnosis.
- *Establishing partnership and trust:*
  - Position yourself as an ally in recovery rather than deferring responsibility to psychiatry.
  - Encourage open dialogue, use visual aids, and provide written resources to reinforce explanations.
- *Providing psychoeducation:*
  - Educate patients about FND symptoms, triggers, and treatment rationale.
  - Emphasize reversibility and the importance of active participation in recovery.

Role of psychoeducation: Psychoeducation reduces stigma, alleviates anxiety, and improves treatment adherence. Patients gain insights into:

- The nature of FND and its symptoms.
- Triggers, maintaining factors, and treatment approaches.
- Strategies for symptom management and relapse prevention.

Benefits:

- Reduces stigma and increases confidence in recovery.
- Reinforces hope and empowers patients to take ownership of their treatment.

WHY COMMUNICATION IS CRUCIAL?

- *Building trust:* Clear explanations help patients feel understood and validated, reducing fears of dismissal.
- *Empowerment:* Validating symptoms while highlighting treatability instills hope and motivates patients.
- *Avoiding alienation:* Poor communication risks disengagement, abandonment of care, and second opinions.

CONCLUSION

A neurological assessment for FND serves as the foundation for both diagnosis and treatment. Effective communication solidifies trust, reinforces the diagnosis, and empowers patients to engage in recovery. By combining validation, education, therapeutic demonstrations, and psychoeducation, clinicians can optimize outcomes and foster long-term treatment adherence.

Q13. Discuss managing functional neurological disorder (FND): A practical approach for individual doctors.

Ans. Managing functional neurological disorder as an individual doctor can feel challenging, especially without access to a multidisciplinary team. However, it is important to know that you can make a real difference by using the biopsychosocial model to address the biological, psychological, and social aspects of the disorder. Medications, such as antidepressants, anxiolytics, and antipsychotics, can also play a supportive role in addressing psychiatric comorbidities, though they are not the primary treatment for FND. Many patients show improvement when symptoms are validated, explained, and treated holistically. With the right approach, even a single physician can provide meaningful care while gradually building connections to strengthen support.

Biopsychosocial model and its importance:

The biopsychosocial model views health and illness as the result of interactions between biological, psychological, and social factors, making it especially relevant to FND. Instead of focusing solely on physical symptoms, it considers how biological factors (e.g., brain function and genetics), psychological factors (e.g., stress and trauma), and social factors (e.g., relationships and environment) influence the disorder. This approach emphasizes understanding the whole patient rather than isolating symptoms, enabling doctors to create personalized treatment plans. By addressing all these dimensions, doctors can improve outcomes even without access to a full team.

Ideal multidisciplinary approach:

In an ideal setting, FND is managed by a team of neurologists, physiotherapists, psychologists, occupational therapists, and social workers. This team approach allows for:

- Comprehensive assessments to address physical, emotional, and social factors
- Rehabilitation programs focused on motor retraining and functional recoveryPsychological support through therapies such as cognitive behavioral therapy (CBT) to manage stress and traumaSocial reintegration strategies, including workplace adjustments and social support

While this model is highly effective, it is not always immediately available, particularly in smaller practices or rural areas. This makes it essential for individual doctors to take the lead in care.

Role of medications—a supportive role, not primary treatment:

Medications such as antidepressants, anxiolytics, and antipsychotics can help manage psychiatric comorbidities such as depression, anxiety, or psychosis, which are common in FND patients. However, they are not effective in treating the core functional symptoms directly and should be used as adjuncts rather than primary treatments.

- *Antidepressants and anxiolytics:* Useful for reducing emotional distress, improving therapy engagement, and addressing coexisting mood disorders.

- *Risks:* Medications may occasionally worsen symptoms (e.g., abnormal movements) or mask underlying organic diseases if used indiscriminately. Careful selection and monitoring are essential.
- *Key consideration:* Prescriptions should complement other therapies and never replace physical or psychological rehabilitation.

Practical steps for individual doctors:
When managing FND without a full team, focus on education, reassurance, and symptom relief:
- *Validate symptoms:*
    - Reassure patients that their symptoms are real and caused by brain function changes, not imagination.
    - Educate them about FND to reduce anxiety and stigma.
- *Address biological factors:*
    - Conduct thorough evaluations to rule out structural causes.
    - Provide medications for associated issues such as migraines, pain, or sleep problems.
    - Recommend physical therapy or graded exercises to improve mobility and motor control.
- *Support psychological health:*
    - Screen for anxiety, depression, and trauma and explain their connection to FND.
    - Introduce basic stress management tools, such as mindfulness and relaxation techniques.
    - Suggest online CBT programs or mental health apps if therapists are unavailable.
- *Build social support:*
    - Engage family members to provide emotional support and reduce isolation.
    - Connect patients with support groups and online communities for shared experiences.
    - Offer practical advice for adapting work routines or daily activities.

Expanding toward a team approach:
Over time, doctors can build partnerships to broaden care:
- *Referral networks:* Connect with neurologists, physiotherapists, and psychologists for specialized help.
- *Telemedicine options:* Use virtual consultations to access distant specialists.
- *Community resources:* Guide patients to charities, advocacy groups, and social workers for additional support.

Key takeaway:
Even without a multidisciplinary team, an individual doctor can manage FND effectively by focusing on education, symptom relief, and patient empowerment. Gradually expanding referral networks and leveraging community resources helps create a more comprehensive approach over time. Medications play a supportive role in managing psychiatric

comorbidities but should not be the primary treatment. With reassurance and practical tools, doctors can offer meaningful care and help patients regain confidence and control over their lives.

Q14. What is the role of the neurologist and the psychiatrist in functional neurological disorders (FND)? Who should assume ownership of the patient? Is the neurologist's job done, when he has made a diagnosis and should he now just send off to a psychiatry colleague? Discuss the roles of the neurologist and the psychiatrist in FND management.

Ans.

INTRODUCTION: EVOLVING ROLE OF THE NEUROLOGIST

Historically, neurologists diagnosed functional neurological disorder (FND) and referred patients to psychiatrists for further management. However, FND management has evolved, highlighting an expanded role for neurologists that extends beyond diagnosis. Patients typically present with neurological symptoms and seek care from neurologists, not psychiatrists. Simply referring them to psychiatry can erode trust, reinforce stigma, and imply their symptoms are "not real." Many patients may not yet accept or understand the psychological aspects of FND. Neurologists must remain actively involved, serving as a bridge to multidisciplinary care and fostering a patient-centered approach.

ROLE OF THE NEUROLOGIST

- *Diagnosis:*
  - Perform a thorough neurological assessment to rule out organic causes.
  - Identify positive signs (e.g., Hoover's sign) to confidently diagnose FND based on findings rather than exclusion.
- *Patient communication:*
  - Provide a clear, empathetic explanation that FND is a real, treatable condition.
  - Educate patients about FND's reversibility and emphasize the importance of active participation in treatment.
- *Management:*
  - Coordinate multidisciplinary care, referring to physiotherapists, psychologists, or occupational therapists as needed.
  - Prescribe symptomatic treatments and address comorbid neurological conditions.
  - Monitor symptoms, reassess treatment, and ensure ongoing patient engagement.

- *Follow-up:*
  - Address symptom progression, provide support, and adjust management strategies.

ROLE OF THE PSYCHIATRIST

- *Assessment:*
  - Evaluate and manage psychological aspects, including depression, anxiety, and PTSD.
  - Assess psychosocial factors contributing to symptoms.
- *Treatment:*
  - Provide therapies such as cognitive-behavioral therapy (CBT) to address coping mechanisms and beliefs.
  - Treat emotional and interpersonal factors affecting symptoms.
- *Collaboration:*
  - Work closely with the neurologist and other specialists to integrate psychiatric and neurological management.

Who Should Assume Ownership?

- *Multidisciplinary care:* Both neurologists and psychiatrists should co-manage patients to address neurological and psychological aspects.
- *Shared model:*
  - Neurologists lead when neurological symptoms predominate.
  - Psychiatrists lead when psychological issues dominate.

Is the Neurologist's Job Done after Diagnosis?

- *No.* The neurologist must:
  - Monitor symptoms, provide follow-up, and coordinate care.
  - Reinforce the legitimacy of FND as a neurological disorder.
  - Prevent stigma by staying involved and avoiding premature psychiatric referrals.

CONCLUSION

Optimal FND management requires collaboration between neurologists and psychiatrists, integrating neurological and psychological expertise. The neurologist's expanded role ensures the patient feels supported, symptoms are legitimized, and they are connected to resources for holistic care. This multidisciplinary approach provides the best chance for positive outcomes and sustained treatment engagement.

Key takeaways:

- *Expanded role of neurologists*—from diagnosis to ongoing care, coordination, and education.
- *Key contributions of psychiatrists*—assessment, therapy, and addressing emotional factors.
- *Multidisciplinary ownership*—shared care between neurologists and psychiatrists.
- *Reinforcement against stigma*—neurologists must stay engaged to build trust and validate symptoms.

Q15. A young man comes with sudden onset weakness of one limb. When do you suspect a functional disorder and how do you differentiate it from limb weakness due to other neurological disorders such as stroke or a plexus lesion (one limb or hemiparesis)?

Ans.

SUDDEN ONSET LIMB WEAKNESS: FUNCTIONAL VERSUS STRUCTURAL CAUSES

When evaluating sudden onset weakness of one limb or hemiparesis in a young person, differentiating functional neurological disorders (FND) from structural neurological causes such as stroke or plexus lesions is crucial. Functional weakness should be suspected when specific clinical features suggest inconsistency or non-anatomical patterns of dysfunction.

When to Suspect Functional Weakness?

- *Inconsistency:*
  - Weakness varies during the examination or between tasks.
- *Distractibility:*
  - Weakness improves when the patient's attention is diverted.
- *Non-physiological Patterns:*
  - Weakness does not align with known anatomical or neurophysiological distributions.
- *Positive functional signs:*
  - Tests such as Hoover's sign (leg weakness) or hip abductor sign can indicate functional weakness.
- *Preserved reflexes and tone:*
  - Despite significant weakness, reflexes and muscle tone remain normal.
- *Associated symptoms:*
  - Presence of other functional symptoms or comorbidities (e.g., fibromyalgia).
- *Precipitating factors:*
  - Recent stress, minor injuries, or psychological distress.

KEY CLINICAL DIFFERENCES (TABLE 1)

TABLE 1: Key clinical differences.

Feature	Functional weakness	Structural weakness
Pattern of weakness	Entire limb uniformly affected	Follows neuroanatomical patterns (e.g., nerve roots, stroke territories)
Onset	Often nonspecific or gradual	Sudden in vascular events; focal in nerve/plexus injuries
Reflexes	Normal	Altered (e.g., hyperreflexia in stroke, reduced in plexus injury)
Associated features	Other functional symptoms	Neurological signs such as sensory level or cranial nerve involvement
Imaging	Normal MRI	May show stroke or plexus abnormality

KEY CLINICAL TESTS

- *Hoover's sign (leg weakness):*
    - *How to perform:* Place one hand under the heel of the unaffected leg and ask the patient to lift the weak leg.
    - *Findings:*
        - *Functional weakness:* No downward pressure felt on the unaffected leg.
        - *Structural weakness:* Downward pressure present as an attempt is made.
- *Pronator drift test (arm weakness):*
    - *How to perform:* Ask the patient to extend both arms forward, palms up, and close their eyes.
    - *Findings:*
        - *Functional weakness:* Inconsistent or absent drift, often improving with distraction.
        - *Structural weakness:* Affected arm drifts downward with pronation.
- *Sensory examination:*
    - Functional weakness may present with non-anatomical sensory changes (e.g., glove-and-stocking patterns).
- *Gait analysis:*
    - Functional hemiparesis may cause a dragging leg gait rather than circumduction typical of stroke.

ROLE OF INVESTIGATIONS

- *Neuroimaging:*
    - Magnetic resonance imaging (MRI) to rule out structural causes such as stroke or plexus lesions.
- *Electrophysiology:*
    - Nerve conduction studies may help in suspected plexus or peripheral nerve lesions.
- *Rule-in features:*
    - Diagnosis of functional weakness is confirmed with positive clinical signs, not just exclusion.

CONCLUSION

Functional limb weakness should be suspected in cases of sudden onset weakness with inconsistent findings, distractibility, and normal neuroimaging. Differentiation relies on clinical signs, patient history, and targeted investigations to rule out structural causes. A multidisciplinary approach ensures accurate diagnosis and management.

Q16. A person comes with jerking movements of limbs and unresponsiveness. When will you suspect functional seizures and what are the clinical clues to differentiate them from epileptic seizures? Discuss the role of investigations, such as electroencephalogram (EEG), video EEG?

Ans.

FUNCTIONAL SEIZURES VERSUS EPILEPTIC SEIZURES

Functional seizures or psychogenic non-epileptic seizures (PNES) mimic epileptic seizures but arise from psychological or functional factors rather than abnormal brain activity. Differentiating the two is critical as management strategies differ, and accurate diagnosis relies on clinical evaluation supported by investigations such as video electroencephalogram (EEG).

When to Suspect Functional Seizures?

Functional seizures should be considered when:

- *Atypical seizure characteristics:* Seizure patterns do not align with known epileptic presentations.
- *Prolonged duration:* Events lasting >5 minutes without significant autonomic changes or post-ictal confusion.
- *High event frequency:* Frequent seizures not responding to anti-epileptic drugs (AEDs).
- *Fluctuating symptoms:* Variability in presentation during or across events.
- *Psychological history:* Evidence of psychological trauma, stress, or functional symptoms.
- *Lack of response to AEDs:* No improvement despite appropriate dosing.

CLINICAL CLUES TO DIFFERENTIATE FUNCTIONAL AND EPILEPTIC SEIZURES (TABLE 2)

TABLE 2: Clinical clues to differentiate functional and epileptic seizures.

Feature	Functional seizures	Epileptic seizures
Onset	Gradual	Sudden
Duration	Often prolonged (>5 minutes)	Typically 1–2 minutes
Termination	Gradual	Abrupt
Eye movement	Closed, resistance to eye opening	Open or closed, no resistance
Motor activity	Asynchronous, out-of-phase movements	Synchronized and stereotypical

Continued

Continued

Feature	Functional seizures	Epileptic seizures
Head movement	Side-to-side common	Tonic deviation
Pelvic thrusting	Common	Rare
Vocalization	Ictal crying/weeping	Guttural cry at onset
Responsiveness	Variable; may follow commands	Usually unresponsive
Injury	Rarely causes serious injuries	Higher risk (burns and tongue biting)
Post-ictal state	Rapid recovery	Prolonged confusion and sleepiness
Autonomic changes	Minimal	Prominent (e.g., tachycardia)
Electroencephalogram (EEG) during event	Normal	Abnormal electrical activity
Triggers	Emotional stress, situational (confirmed)	Consistent (e.g., sleep deprivation)

ROLE OF INVESTIGATIONS

- *Routine electroencephalogram:*
  - Normal ictal EEG during events supports functional seizures.
  - Interictal epileptiform discharges suggest epilepsy but are not definitive.
- *Video electroencephalogram:*
  - *Gold standard:* Correlates semiology with EEG findings.
  - Absence of ictal EEG changes during typical events confirms functional seizures.
- *Prolactin levels:*
  - Elevated levels post-ictally support epilepsy but lack specificity for routine use.
- *Neuroimaging (magnetic resonance imaging):*
  - Rules out structural causes but is not essential for functional seizure diagnosis.
- *Psychological assessment:*
  - Identifies underlying stress, trauma, or psychosocial contributors.

Key Considerations

- *Combination of features:* No single feature can definitively differentiate functional seizures from epileptic seizures. A combination of clinical and investigative findings is required.
- *Reliable signs:* Ictal eye closure and asynchronous limb movements are particularly useful for identifying functional seizures.

- *Comorbidity:* Functional seizures and epilepsy can coexist in 10–30% of cases, complicating the diagnostic process.
- *Multidisciplinary approach:* Neurologists, epileptologists, psychiatrists, and psychologists are integral to comprehensive management.

CONCLUSION

The diagnosis of functional seizures relies on recognizing specific "rule-in" features through clinical observation and investigations, particularly video EEG. Functional seizures demand a multidisciplinary care model addressing both neurological and psychological aspects. Early recognition and effective communication of the diagnosis are critical for optimal management and improved patient outcomes.

Q17. What are functional sensory symptoms generally seen in clinical practice? How to recognize whether they are functional or organic? Are there any patterns in sensory loss indicative of functional sensory disorders?

Ans. Functional sensory symptoms are sensory disturbances without an identifiable organic or structural cause. They often defy neuroanatomical or physiological explanations and require a detailed clinical approach for accurate recognition and diagnosis.

Common functional sensory symptoms are as follows:

- *Numbness*: Reported as complete or partial loss of sensation
- *Tingling or pins-and-needles*: Diffuse or localized, inconsistent with dermatomal distributions
- *Temperature sensations*: Altered perception of heat or cold in non-anatomical patterns.
- *Sensory loss*: Does not align with nerve or dermatome pathways, often described as "glove-and-stocking" or unilateral whole-limb sensory loss

How to recognize functional versus organic sensory symptoms:

- *Inconsistency*:
  - Symptoms vary across examinations or within the same session.
  - Boundaries of sensory loss shift and do not conform to expected neurological pathways
- *Nonanatomical patterns*:
  - Glove-and-stocking sensory loss
  - Whole-limb sensory deficits that ignore nerve root or peripheral nerve distributions
- *Positive neurological signs*:
  - Sensory symptoms that appear incongruent with expected findings
  - Normal reflexes and motor function despite reported sensory loss

- *Psychological context*:
  - History of recent stress, trauma, or psychological distress
  - Symptoms often coincide with emotional or psychosocial challenges.
- *Behavioral observations*:
  - Lack of functional impairment despite reported severe sensory loss
  - Inconsistent reactions during sensory mapping

Patterns suggestive of functional sensory disorders:
- *Unilateral glove-and-stocking sensory loss*: It encompasses the entire hand or foot, not following anatomical pathways.
- *Nondermatomal distribution*: It does not match peripheral nerve or spinal root distributions.
- *Inconsistent findings*: These vary across time or under different conditions.
- *Noncorrelative changes*: These do not correspond with known neurological pathways.

Diagnostic approach:
- *Detailed neurological examination*:
  - Sensory mapping and provocation tests to assess boundaries
  - Compare subjective reports with objective findings
- *Rule-out organic causes*:
  - Neuroimaging and electrophysiological studies (e.g., nerve conduction, somatosensory-evoked potentials)
- *Rule-in features*:
  - Focus on patterns characteristic of functional disorders, not merely the absence of organic findings

Management strategies:
- *Therapeutic alliance*:
  - Build trust and provide clear, empathetic explanations about the condition.
- *Rehabilitation*:
  - Gradual retraining of sensory perception and functional restoration
- *Psychological support*:
  - Address underlying stressors or trauma through cognitive–behavioral therapy.
- *Avoid over-investigation*:
  - Limit unnecessary tests to prevent reinforcing symptom focus.

CONCLUSION

Functional sensory symptoms present distinct, nonanatomical patterns such as inconsistent glove-and-stocking loss or shifting sensory deficits. Diagnosis relies on identifying characteristic positive signs while ruling out organic causes. Management requires a compassionate, multidisciplinary approach that integrates neurological and psychological care to optimize outcomes.

Q18. When do you suspect a functional disorder in an unconscious patient presenting to the emergency department? How do you manage it?

Ans. A functional disorder should be suspected in an unconscious patient presenting to the emergency department when clinical features and examination findings are inconsistent with structural or metabolic causes of coma. Functional coma, also referred to as psychogenic unresponsiveness or dissociative stupor, occurs without structural brain damage or metabolic abnormalities and is often triggered by psychological stress, trauma, or underlying psychiatric conditions. It is more common in young females, especially those with a history of psychiatric illness or recent emotional stressors.

Clues suggesting functional disorder are as follows:

- *Pupillary reactions*: Normal pupillary reflexes despite apparent unresponsiveness; structural causes may cause asymmetric, pinpoint, or sluggish pupils, while metabolic causes may lead to dilated or constricted pupils.
- *Breathing patterns*: Rapid, shallow breathing is typical of functional coma, whereas structural or metabolic causes show patterns like Cheyne–Stokes or Kussmaul respiration.
- *Neurological reflexes*: Functional coma preserves normal tendon reflexes, flexor plantar responses, and corneal reflexes, unlike structural or metabolic coma, where reflexes may be absent, sluggish, or asymmetric.
- *Resistance to eye opening*: Patients with functional disorders often *actively resist eye opening*, whereas organic causes lack muscle tone, allowing passive opening.
- *Absence of trauma signs*: Functional cases typically lack tongue biting, incontinence, or injuries that are more common in structural causes.
- *Positive signs of inconsistency*: Functional patients may:
    - Prevent a paralyzed arm from falling onto their face.
    - Avoid injury by controlling leg drop during testing.
    - React to noxious stimuli like a vibrating tuning fork on the nasal mucosa despite being unresponsive to other painful stimuli.

The comparison with organic causes is given in **Table 3**.

TABLE 3: Comparison with organic causes.

Feature	Functional coma	Structural/metabolic coma
Pupillary reactions	Normal pupillary reflexes	May be sluggish, asymmetric, pinpoint, dilated, or constricted
Breathing patterns	Shallow, rapid respiratory rate	Deep, labored, or irregular (Cheyne–Stokes, Kussmaul)
Reflexes	Normal tendon reflexes and flexor plantar response	Reflexes may be asymmetrical (structural) or sluggish (metabolic)

Continued

Continued

Feature	Functional coma	Structural/metabolic coma
Signs of injury	No incontinence, tongue biting, or trauma	Often associated with injuries, incontinence, or tongue bites
Response to stimuli	May resist arm drop onto face or leg drop onto shin	No voluntary movement; may respond only to deep painful stimuli
Eye opening	Passive resistance to eye opening	No resistance; eyes open easily due to reduced muscle tone
Response to noxious stimuli	Reacts to a vibrating tuning fork on nasal mucosa	Unresponsive to noxious stimuli or shows withdrawal reflex only

The investigations to rule out organic causes are as follows:
- *Neuroimaging [computed tomography (CT)/magnetic resonance imaging (MRI)]*: To exclude stroke, tumors, or structural damage
- *EEG*: Functional coma shows normal activity, whereas structural causes may exhibit suppression or epileptiform discharges.
- *Blood tests*: Assess glucose, electrolytes, and toxins to rule out metabolic causes.

Management: Once a functional diagnosis is confirmed, management focuses on supportive care and addressing psychological factors:
- *Reassurance and explanation*: Clearly explain to the patient and family that the symptoms are real but reversible. This reduces fear, stigma, and anxiety.
- *Psychological support*: Cognitive behavioral therapy (CBT) or psychiatric evaluation to address underlying stressors
- *Physical care*: Maintain hydration, nutrition, and physical safety while monitoring recovery.
- *Avoid reinforcing symptoms*: Encourage gradual mobilization and avoid excessive investigations that may reinforce illness behavior.

Prognosis: Functional coma often resolves quickly with reassurance and supportive therapy. Early identification and intervention improve recovery and reduce recurrence. Long-term management may involve psychiatric follow-up to address stressors and prevent relapse.

Q19. What would make you suspect a functional gait disorder (FGD) in patient with altered gait?

Ans. Functional gait disorders are relatively common, but their diagnosis can be challenging due to the absence of a single defining pattern and overlap with organic gait disorders. Typical presentations include difficulty walking due to apparent weakness, buckling knees, excessive sway, exaggerated effort, a bouncy or scissoring gait, a wide-based stance, or recurrent falls without significant injuries.

However, the hallmark features that point to FGD are inconsistency and incongruency.

- *Inconsistency*:
  - Fluctuating presentation: Gait abnormalities may vary during observation, with patients sometimes walking almost normally outside the clinic while demonstrating significant gait impairment during examination.
  - Mismatch in functionality: Patients may report severe gait problems yet perform daily activities with minimal issues. Conversely, some may overstate their symptoms without observable functional deficits.
  - Variable performance: Family members might describe walking difficulties as inconsistent or changing over time.
- *Incongruency*:
  - Unusual symptom combinations: Signs and symptoms incompatible with known organic disorders; examples include:
    - Buckling knees despite preserved quadriceps power
    - Scissoring gait without increased tone in thigh adductors
    - Ataxic gait with the ability to perform tandem walking (heel-to-toe) smoothly
  - Surprising abilities: During tandem walking, patients might show exaggerated sway or windmill-like arm movements, giving the impression of instability, yet complete the task without sidestepping or falling.

Diagnosis and approach: Clinicians rely on their experience and knowledge of the patient's history to identify FGD. If the diagnosis is uncertain, keeping it open and conducting a re-evaluation later is prudent. The absence of structural or neurological abnormalities on imaging can support the diagnosis. Prompt recognition and management of FGD, emphasizing clear communication and avoiding unnecessary investigations, ensure better outcomes and patient trust.

Understanding the broader context: Patients with FGD often present with emotional or psychological stressors that manifest physically. This highlights the importance of a multidisciplinary approach, including physical therapy, psychological support, and patient education, to address the root causes of the disorder. Early diagnosis reduces unnecessary interventions and sets the stage for effective rehabilitation.

By focusing on the characteristic features of inconsistency and incongruency, clinicians can confidently differentiate FGD from organic disorders, ensuring appropriate care and reassurance for patients.

Q20. What is persistent postural perceptual dizziness (PPPD)? What are its presenting symptoms? How is it diagnosed? What is its pathophysiology? When should we consider the diagnosis of PPPD in patients presenting with dizziness?

Ans. Persistent postural perceptual dizziness is among the most common causes of chronic dizziness. It is a functional neuro-otological disorder characterized by chronic dizziness, imbalance, and hypersensitivity to motion and visual stimuli. It commonly follows vestibular insults like benign paroxysmal positional vertigo (BPPV) or vestibular neuritis, vasovagal syncope, psychological stressors, or migraines, affecting quality of life through persistent symptoms and postural instability.

The presenting symptoms are as follows:

- *Chronic dizziness*:
  - Persistent for ≥3 months on ≥50% of days
  - Described as nonspinning vertigo, unsteadiness, or environmental instability
- *Trigger sensitivity*:
  - Symptoms worsen with:
    - Upright postures (e.g., standing, walking)
    - Motion or visually complex environments
- *Associated features*:
  - Cognitive difficulties during motion-related activities
  - Anticipatory anxiety or hypervigilance
  - Balance disturbances without vertigo

Pathophysiology: PPPD arises from maladaptive central nervous system changes:

- *Central vestibular dysfunction*:
  - Hyperactivation of cortical vestibular areas disrupts balance and sensory integration.
- *Neuroplasticity*:
  - Chronic symptoms reflect maladaptive recalibration of sensory inputs after a trigger.
- *Neurochemical dysregulation*:
  - Altered serotonergic and noradrenergic pathways amplify sensory sensitivity and anxiety.

Diagnostic criteria: Modified Bárány criteria include:

- *Duration*: Persistent dizziness or unsteadiness ≥3 months
- *Frequency*: Symptoms present ≥50% of days.
- *Triggers*: Symptoms worsen with posture, walking, or visual motion.
- *Exclusion*: Normal imaging and no alternative explanation for symptoms

When to suspect PPPD?

Consider PPPD in patients with:

- Persistent dizziness for over 3 months
- Symptoms exacerbated by posture or motion-rich environments
- A history of vestibular events, stress, or migraines
- Normal vestibular imaging and electrophysiological findings

Management:

- *Vestibular rehabilitation*:
  - Exercises to recalibrate vestibular and sensory systems
- *Cognitive behavioral therapy (CBT)*:
  - Addresses anticipatory anxiety and maladaptive thought patterns
- *Pharmacological treatment*:
  - Selective serotonin reuptake inhibitors (SSRIs) or serotonin and norepinephrine reuptake inhibitors (SNRIs) for neurochemical regulation
- *Psychoeducation*:
  - Enhances patient understanding and engagement

CONCLUSION

PPPD presents as chronic dizziness with a specific symptom pattern and central vestibular dysfunction. A thorough diagnostic approach and multidisciplinary management can effectively alleviate symptoms and improve quality of life.

Q21. What are functional movement disorders (FMDs) and how to suspect them?

Ans. Functional movement disorders are abnormal involuntary movements that lack a structural or neurodegenerative cause and are classified as a subtype of functional neurological disorders (FNDs). These disorders often arise due to dysfunction in brain networks controlling voluntary movements, influenced by psychological factors rather than anatomical damage. Importantly, FMDs are potentially reversible with appropriate diagnosis and treatment.

How to suspect FMDs?

- *Abrupt onset*:
  - Symptoms often appear suddenly without a gradual progression, unlike organic movement disorders.
- *Variability and fluctuation*:
  - Movements may change in frequency, amplitude, or direction over time and often improve with distraction or suggestion.
- *Distractibility and suggestibility*:
  - Symptoms may reduce or disappear during distraction tasks or rhythm tests, such as entrainment.

- *Incongruence with neurological patterns*:
  - Movements do not follow known neuroanatomical pathways or recognized patterns of the known movement disorders.
- *Specific signs and patterns*:
  - Functional tremor: Variable frequency, sudden onset, and entrainment
  - Functional dystonia: Fixed or variable postures, triggered by trauma, often inconsistent

Core features to look for are:

- *Inconsistency*: Symptoms vary depending on tasks or distraction.
- *Incongruity*: Movements contradict expected neurophysiological patterns.
- *Psychological overlay*: Symptoms are often linked to stress, anxiety, or trauma.

Pitfalls and challenges in diagnosis: Certain organic movement disorders, such as dystonia and tics, can resemble functional disorders due to their unusual appearance, variability, and partial suppressibility. For example:

- *Dystonia*: Some forms may have variability and suppressibility, making them appear functional.
- *Tics*: These can be abrupt, bizarre, and influenced by stress, mimicking functional patterns.
- *Parkinsonian tremor*: May vary with posture and mimic functional tremor

How to avoid misdiagnosis?

- *Detailed history and examination*:
  - Focus on onset, progression, triggers, and associated psychological factors.
- *Rule-in positive features of FMDs*:
  - Use tests such as Hoover's sign or entrainment to identify functional characteristics.
- *Neurophysiological testing*:
  - Use electromyography (EMG), video recordings, and tremor analysis to evaluate patterns of muscle activation.
- *Second opinion or specialist referral*:
  - Refer to neurologists specializing in movement disorders for complex cases.
- *Longitudinal observation*:
  - Monitor symptoms over time to distinguish fixed patterns of organic disorders from fluctuating features of FMDs.

Management and prognosis: FMDs are often treatable with multidisciplinary approaches, including:

- *Psychoeducation*: Helping patients understand the diagnosis
- *Physiotherapy and motor retraining*: Addressing movement patterns and functional restoration
- *Cognitive behavioral therapy (CBT)*: Managing psychological contributors
- *Prognosis*: Favorable outcomes are achievable with early diagnosis and intervention.

CONCLUSION

FMDs are characterized by abrupt onset, variability, distractibility, and incongruence with organic patterns. However, some organic disorders like dystonia and tics may appear functional due to their variability and suppressibility. Clinicians should carefully assess positive features, use neurophysiological tests, and seek specialist input when needed to avoid misdiagnosis and optimize management.

Q22. When to suspect functional tremors and how to prove it?

Ans. Functional tremors are the most common subtype of functional movement disorders (FMDs), accounting for up to 50% of cases. These tremors often mimic organic tremors but display distinctive characteristics that help in diagnosis.

The key features of functional tremors are as follows:

- *Inconsistent tremor phenomenology*:
    - Tremors display variability in amplitude and frequency across tasks.
    - Tremors may change characteristics or cease entirely with distraction.
    - Symptoms worsen with attention and improve with distraction, opposite to organic tremors.
- *Incongruent features*:
    - Tremors do not follow neuroanatomical or neurophysiological patterns.
    - Movements may appear exaggerated or performative.
    - Variability across different body parts or examination conditions

Diagnostic signs to prove functional tremors are mentioned in **Table 4**.

TABLE 4: Diagnostic signs to prove functional tremors.

Sign name	Technique	Interpretation
Whack-a-mole sign	Suppress tremor in one limb and observe if it shifts to another body part	Indicates nonorganic origin with variability and psychological influence
Entrainment sign	Ask the patient to tap rhythmically with the opposite hand or foot. Observe changes in tremor rhythm	Tremors often synchronize with rhythmic movement or disappear entirely
Distractibility test	Engage the patient in cognitive tasks (counting backward, spelling words). Monitor tremor response	Tremor diminishes or disappears under cognitive load, suggesting functional origin
Magnification sign	Observe tremor casually, then explicitly measure it to see if symptoms amplify with attention	Tremor amplitude increases when focus is drawn, highlighting psychological factors
Variability sign	Observe tremor across multiple scenarios—sitting, standing, with eyes open/closed	Tremor characteristics change dramatically in frequency, amplitude, or distribution across different conditions

Differentiating functional from common organic tremors:
- *Parkinson's tremor:*
  - Appears at rest, reduces with voluntary movement, and reemerges during posture-holding
  - Consistent and predictable, typically starting asymmetrically (unilateral) before becoming bilateral
  - Often associated with rigidity and bradykinesia
- *Essential tremor:*
  - Bilateral, symmetric, and primarily occurs during action (postural or kinetic).
  - Consistent frequency across tasks and improves temporarily with alcohol.
  - Absent at rest, unlike functional or Parkinson's tremors
  - May be long-standing or have a family history
- *Functional tremor:*
  - Can be abrupt in onset
  - Highly variable in frequency, amplitude, and distribution
  - Improves with distraction, shows entrainment, and lacks predictable patterns.
  - May shift between limbs or cease entirely under observation

Neurophysiological testing: Electromyography (EMG) and accelerometry can help identify irregular patterns inconsistent with organic tremors.

Treatment approaches: These include psychoeducation, physiotherapy with motor retraining, and cognitive behavioral therapy (CBT).

Prognosis: Favorable with early diagnosis and intervention.

CONCLUSION

Functional tremors are the most common type of FMDs and differ significantly from Parkinson's and essential tremors. Functional tremors show variability, distractibility, and incongruence with organic patterns. Positive signs like entrainment and distractibility help confirm diagnosis. Distinguishing them from organic tremors requires careful assessment, neurophysiological testing, and timely intervention to ensure better outcomes.

Q23. What are the key features of functional parkinsonism, and how does it differ from idiopathic Parkinson's disease (PD)?

Ans. Functional parkinsonism is a subtype of functional neurological disorder (FND) that mimics idiopathic PD but differs in key features. Functional parkinsonism accounts for 3–5% of all FMDs and <1.5% of all parkinsonism cases. It is typically nonprogressive and potentially reversible.

The key clinical features of functional parkinsonism are as follows:
- *Symptom onset and progression:*
  - Abrupt onset, often following stress or trauma

 - Symptoms remain stable without progression, unlike the gradual worsening seen in PD.
- *Tremor patterns*:
 - Tremor is present in all positions (rest, posture, kinetic), unlike PD, which primarily involves resting tremor.
 - Tremor amplitude decreases with distraction or entrainment and lacks reemergence seen in PD.
- *Rigidity and movement abnormalities*:
 - Absence of cogwheel rigidity; instead, there is oppositional stiffness that disappears with distraction.
 - Slowness (bradykinesia) without reduced amplitude, unlike PD, which shows decrementing movements
- *Gait and posture abnormalities*:
 - Exaggerated arm swing or flailing movements with disproportionate slowness
 - Unusual gait patterns like astasia–abasia or buckling knees, not typical of PD.
- *Speech and associated features*:
 - Speech changes such as whispering, stuttering, or gibberish speech
 - Excessive effortful behaviors like grunting or sighing (e.g., "huffing and puffing" sign)

Key differences between functional parkinsonism and idiopathic PD are mentioned in **Table 5**.

TABLE 5: Key differences between functional parkinsonism and idiopathic Parkinson's disease.

Feature	Functional parkinsonism	Idiopathic Parkinson's disease
Onset	Sudden, often linked to stress or trauma	Gradual, progressive worsening over time
Tremor	Present in all states (rest, posture, kinetic); suppressible by distraction	Resting tremor that improves with action and reemerges with posture
Rigidity	Oppositional stiffness without cogwheel rigidity	Cogwheel rigidity with consistent resistance during passive movement
Bradykinesia	Slowness without decrement in movement amplitude	Progressive reduction in movement amplitude (decrementing movements)
Gait patterns	Astasia–abasia, exaggerated responses, buckling knees	Shuffling gait, stooped posture, reduced arm swing
Speech	Whispering, stuttering, effortful speech (psychogenic features)	Hypophonia, monotone, slow speech
Response to dopaminergic therapy	Poor or absent response	Significant improvement with dopamine therapy
Neuroimaging	Normal nigrostriatal function on PET/SPECT	Abnormal striatal dopamine uptake patterns

(PET: positron emission tomography; SPECT: single-photon emission computed tomography)

Investigations:

- *Electromyography (EMG)*: To evaluate tremor variability and entrainment patterns.
- *TRODAT or DaTSCAN imaging*: Functional parkinsonism shows normal nigrostriatal dopamine function, unlike PD.

Management and prognosis:

- *Treatment approaches*:
  - Psychoeducation to explain the diagnosis positively
  - Cognitive behavioral therapy (CBT) for associated psychological triggers
  - Physiotherapy and motor retraining for movement normalization
- *Prognosis*: Favorable with multidisciplinary interventions and early diagnosis

CONCLUSION

Functional parkinsonism can mimic idiopathic PD but demonstrates variability, distractibility, and inconsistencies. Differentiating it from PD relies on clinical signs, neurophysiological tests, and imaging studies. Early recognition and treatment improve outcomes, highlighting the importance of positive communication and a patient-centered approach.

Q24. A person comes with intermittent abnormal movements. How do you distinguish functional ones from paroxysmal dystonia or chorea?

Ans. Functional paroxysmal movement disorders are a subtype of functional neurological disorders (FNDs) characterized by intermittent abnormal movements that lack an organic basis. They can mimic paroxysmal dystonia or chorea but differ in clinical presentation, triggers, and response patterns.

Key features of functional paroxysmal movement disorders are as follows:

- *Phenomenological variability*: High variability between episodes, unlike paroxysmal kinesigenic dyskinesia (PKD), which shows stereotyped, repetitive movements.
- *Mixed presentations*: Combinations of dystonia, tremors, and jerks, often involving multiple body parts
- *Symmetry*: Bilateral limb involvement is common, whereas PKD is often unilateral.
- *Trigger and duration*: Atypical and variable triggers, durations, and severity of episodes
- *Suggestibility*: Movements may worsen with suggestion or examination.
- *Altered responsiveness*: Changes in consciousness or responsiveness during episodes
- *Unusual relieving maneuvers*: Specific but unusual ways to terminate or modify episodes

Supporting features for functional diagnosis are mentioned here:

- *Psychogenic signs*: Co-occurrence of other medically unexplained symptoms
- *Medication response*: Poor response to most medications, but partial response to benzodiazepines or placebo
- *Somatization features*: Presence of somatic complaints and heightened focus on symptoms
- *Precipitation during examination*: Attacks often precipitated or worsened during testing
- *Paroxysmal tremor association*: Tremor often observed as a predominant feature.

Distinguishing from organic disorders:

- *PKD*: Stereotyped, brief episodes, often triggered by sudden movements
- *Chorea*: Continuous, flowing, nonpatterned movements without distractibility
- *Dystonia*: Fixed, patterned postures with predictable triggers

Management:

- *Multidisciplinary approach*: Education, physiotherapy, and cognitive behavioral therapy (CBT)
- *Prognosis*: Favorable outcomes with early diagnosis and treatment

CONCLUSION

Functional paroxysmal disorders differ from organic causes based on variability, distractibility, and atypical patterns. Clear diagnosis using positive signs and tailored treatment approaches ensures better outcomes.

Q25. A lady comes with sudden-onset vision loss. What are the clues to diagnose functional vision loss or functional blindness?

Ans. When a patient presents with sudden vision loss, distinguishing between functional vision loss and organic causes is crucial. Functional vision loss arises from psychological or functional disruptions rather than structural damage and requires a thorough, empathetic evaluation combining neurological, ophthalmological, and psychological insights.

Clues to functional vision loss are mentioned here:

- *Visual field patterns*:
  - Functional: Tubular or keyhole-shaped fields that remain consistent regardless of testing distance
  - Organic: Visual fields follow neuroanatomical patterns, such as quadrant or hemianopia.
- *Neurological examination*:
  - Functional:
    - Optokinetic nystagmus (OKN): Intact, suggesting preserved unconscious visual processing
    - Consensual pupillary reflexes: Normal in functional monocular blindness.

    - Organic: Absent or abnormal reflexes in severe optic nerve or retinal pathology
- *Behavioral observations*:
    - Functional: Patients may unconsciously navigate spaces well, showing preserved spatial awareness despite reported blindness.
    - Organic: Navigation is typically impaired according to the degree of vision loss.
- *Testing for functional signs*:
    - Mirror test: Functional blindness may allow recognition of reflection despite reported inability to see.
    - Prism adaptation: Patients may unconsciously adapt to visual distortions introduced by a prism lens.
    - Ishihara color plates: Inconsistent or dramatically impaired color vision suggests functional causes.
- *Psychological context*:
    - Functional: History of recent stress, trauma, or conversion disorder indicators
    - Organic: May have secondary psychological impacts but lacks primary stress-related triggers

Diagnostic investigations are given as follows:
- *Neuroimaging*:
    - Functional: Normal magnetic resonance imaging (MRI) with no structural abnormalities
    - Organic: Structural lesions (e.g., optic nerve atrophy, ischemia) on imaging
- *Visual-evoked potentials (VEP)*:
    - Functional: Normal responses, reflecting intact signal transmission
    - Organic: Delayed or absent responses in optic nerve or visual pathway damage
- *Electroretinography (ERG)*:
    - Functional: Normal retinal responses
    - Organic: Abnormal findings in retinal pathologies

The key features to differentiate between functional and organic vision loss are mentioned in **Table 6**.

TABLE 6: Key features to differentiate between functional and organic vision loss.

Dimension	Functional vision loss	Organic vision loss
Field defects	Irregular, nonanatomical	Follows neuroanatomical pathways
Pupillary reflexes	Normal	Impaired in optic nerve/retinal pathology
Navigation	Inconsistent, paradoxical visual competence	Consistent impairment
Imaging	Normal	Structural abnormalities
Neurophysiology (VEP)	Normal	Abnormal
Triggers	Recent stress or psychological trauma	Pathological or vascular origin

Management approach:

- *Multidisciplinary assessment*:
  - Ophthalmologist for detailed ocular examination
  - Neurologist for ruling out structural causes
  - Mental health professional for evaluating psychological contributors
- *Therapeutic interventions*:
  - Psychoeducation: Explain functional vision loss empathetically to foster understanding and engagement.
  - Cognitive behavioral therapy (CBT): Address underlying psychological factors.
  - Gradual rehabilitation: Reinforce visual confidence through structured exercises.

CONCLUSION

Functional vision loss is a genuine condition requiring a careful balance of clinical expertise, empathetic communication, and targeted testing. By integrating neurological, ophthalmological, and psychological perspectives, clinicians can provide accurate diagnoses and comprehensive care, addressing both the visual symptoms and their underlying causes.

Q26. A 24-year-old male presented with bizarre eye movements in the form of sudden onset, persistence convergence of both eyes so that it appeared that he was looking toward tip of nose. Can these abnormal eye movements be functional? What are the functional eye movement disorders (FEMDs) and how to approach them?

Ans. Yes, these abnormal eye movements can be functional. FEMDs are a subtype of functional neurological disorders (FNDs), which affect voluntary eye movements without any structural or neurological damage. Importantly, FEMDs are rarely the presenting symptom but are often detected incidentally during neurological examinations, particularly in patients being evaluated for other functional disorders like gait abnormalities, tremors, or dizziness.

Functional eye movement disorders:

- *Functional convergence spasm*: This is the most common FEMD, characterized by sustained convergence of both eyes, mimicking fixation on a near object. It may resemble sixth cranial nerve palsy due to apparent difficulty in abducting the eyes. However, the presence of variability, miosis (pupillary constriction) and improvement with distraction differentiates it from organic causes.
- *Functional eye oscillations*: These resemble ocular flutter with rapid, brief (2–5 seconds) to-and-fro movements, often confined to the horizontal plane. They may decrease in intensity with repeated testing and can occur alongside head tremors.

- *Functional diplopia*: Unlike organic diplopia, functional diplopia may be monocular and persists even when the unaffected eye is closed. It often lacks anatomical correlation and may fluctuate during examination.
- *Other FEMDs*: Functional gaze paralysis, tonic eye deviation, voluntary nystagmus, and functional opsoclonus may also be observed, often during eye movement testing rather than as the primary complaint.

Approach to diagnosis:
- *Clinical testing*: Assess variability, distractibility, and inconsistencies during examination. Movements often improve with distraction or suggestion.
- *Reflexive testing*: Optokinetic nystagmus or doll's eye responses are typically preserved, differentiating FEMDs from organic causes.
- *Imaging and electrophysiology*: These are used only to exclude organic pathology when needed. FEMDs are diagnosed by positive clinical signs rather than exclusion alone.
- *Video documentation*: It helps to capture inconsistencies for analysis and patient education.

Management: Treatment focuses on a multidisciplinary approach:
- *Education and reassurance*: Explain the diagnosis clearly, emphasizing that symptoms are real but reversible, reducing fear and stigma.
- *Cognitive behavioral therapy (CBT)*: It addresses underlying stressors or anxiety contributing to symptoms.
- *Eye exercises and rehabilitation*: Gradual retraining of movements to restore function
- *Holistic care*: It includes physiotherapy and mental health interventions to treat associated functional symptoms.

Prognosis: With early recognition and intervention, FEMDs often respond well to therapy. Since they are frequently discovered incidentally rather than being the primary complaint, addressing underlying functional disorders through patient education, validation of symptoms, and structured therapy improves both recovery and quality of life.

Q27. When a patient comes with memory loss or other cognitive symptoms how does one suspect a functional disorder versus a degenerative dementia?

Ans. Functional cognitive disorder (FCD) accounts for a significant percentage (12–56%) of referrals to memory clinics and often mimics early Alzheimer's disease or other forms of dementia. Patients commonly report subjective memory complaints, leading to concerns about degenerative disorders. However, FCD differs fundamentally in mechanisms, prognosis, and diagnostic features. Distinguishing FCD from neurodegenerative conditions is critical to avoid misdiagnosis, unnecessary investigations, and inappropriate treatments. Sometimes the memory loss can be acute in onset.

How to suspect a functional disorder?

- *Clinical presentation*:
  - Symptoms are often inconsistent and fluctuating, improving with distraction or focus shifts.
  - Patients report vivid and detailed memory lapses, which are disproportionate to objective findings.
  - Functional abilities are typically preserved, despite complaints of severe cognitive impairment.
  - Symptoms may worsen under stress or fatigue, suggesting psychological influence.
- *Behavioral clues*:
  - Patients may show heightened emotional responses and over-focus on symptoms.
  - Effort during testing can appear excessive or inconsistent, often improving with reassurance.
  - Memory problems may involve specific periods or emotionally charged events, unlike global deficits seen in dementia.
- *Cognitive testing results*:
  - Functional disorders exhibit variable performance, influenced by attention and effort.
  - Delayed recall is often better than immediate recall, which is inconsistent with dementia.
  - Degenerative dementias demonstrate predictable, progressive deficits and decline.
- *Neuroimaging findings*:
  - FCD patients typically have normal structural imaging, while dementia often shows atrophy or structural abnormalities.

Acute amnesia: Functional versus organic causes:

- *Functional acute amnesia*:
  - Triggered by stress or emotional trauma
  - Memory loss is selective for events rather than generalized.
  - Procedural memory and orientation remain intact.
- *Organic acute amnesia*:
  - Associated with structural lesions like stroke or Wernicke's encephalopathy
  - Presents with consistent memory deficits and associated signs (e.g., aphasia or disorientation)
  - Confirmed by neuroimaging showing localized damage

In both situations the key diagnostic marker is internal inconsistency:

- Functional patients may struggle with formal tests but perform well in casual interactions.
- Memory recall varies across contexts, often improving with distraction.
- Positive signs such as preserved recall during indirect questioning support a functional diagnosis.

Comparative table: Cognitive disorders differentiation is given in **Table 7**.

TABLE 7: Cognitive disorders differentiation.

Feature	FCD	Dementia
Cognitive performance	Variable, inconsistent	Progressive, consistent decline
Neuropsychological testing	Effort-dependent, fluctuating	Predictable deficits
Neuroimaging	Normal structure	Atrophy, regional loss
Progression	Nonprogressive, reversible	Progressive deterioration
Psychological influence	High	Minimal
Memory features	Inconsistent, context-dependent	Consistent, progressive loss
Functional impact	Minimal	Significant decline
Treatment approach	CBT, psychological therapy	Symptomatic, supportive care
Prognosis	Reversible	Progressive

(FCD: functional cognitive disorder; CBT: cognitive behavioral therapy)

Functional cognitive disorder can closely mimic degenerative dementia, making careful evaluation crucial. Functional symptoms are often inconsistent, stress-related, and reversible, contrasting with the progressive nature of dementia. Clinicians should focus on positive diagnostic signs, neuropsychological patterns, and imaging findings to differentiate FCD confidently. Early recognition and reassurance, coupled with education, cognitive-behavioral therapy, and stress management, provide the best outcomes while minimizing misdiagnosis and unnecessary treatments.

Q28. A 65-year-old patient present with acute-onset inability to speak. He can understand all spoken and written words but is unable to speak clearly. Can it be functional? What are functional disorders of voice and speech?

Ans. Functional voice and speech disorders (FVSDs) are common neurological presentations across all age-groups, characterized by symptoms without structural abnormalities. Diagnosis is based on recognizing distinctive clinical features and positive diagnostic signs that differentiate them from organic conditions.

Key diagnostic features and red flags:

- *Suggestibility*: Symptoms change with attention or suggestion.
- *Distractibility*: Speech improves with distraction.
- *Acute onset*: Sudden symptoms without clear causes
- *Variability*: Fluctuating severity across tasks
- *Paradoxical muscle response*: Increased tension with fatigue
- *Reversibility*: Potential for rapid improvement

- *Emotional response*: Indifference or denial of symptoms
- *Paradoxical vocal cord movements*: Abnormal patterns on laryngoscopy

Functional voice disorders (FVDs): Common presentations include:
- *Aphonia/dysphonia*: Loss of voice, whispering, or strained voice with normal laryngeal anatomy
- *Puberphonia*: Persistent high-pitched voice, often in adolescents
- *Globus sensation*: Feeling of a lump in the throat without structural cause; diagnosis relies on symptom inconsistency, normal laryngoscopy, and improvement with distraction or tasks like laughing.

Functional speech disorders (FSDs): FSD affects articulation, fluency, or prosody:
- *Stuttering*: Stress-induced and variable
- *Rhythmic/prosodic issues*: Hypernasality, altered pitch, broken patterns
- *Functional foreign accent syndrome*: Variable accents and improvement with distraction
- *Articulation abnormalities*: Inconsistent errors, paradoxical tongue movements, and give-way weakness

Differentiation from organic disorders: Functional disorders differ from aphasia and dysarthria:
- *Onset*: Functional symptoms are sudden, inconsistent, and fluctuating.
- *Automatic speech*: Preserved fluency with tasks like singing or counting
- *Imaging*: Normal structural findings
- *Response to distraction*: Improvement with focus shifts
- *Emotional response*: Indifference (la belle indifférence) versus frustration in organic cases
- *Neurological examination*: Functional cases show incongruent findings; organic cases align with lesion sites.

Diagnosis and management: The diagnosis of FVD or FSD relies on ruling in functional features such as variability, distractibility, and incongruence with organic patterns, supported by detailed clinical examination and imaging. Key steps include:
1. Patient reassurance and explanation to establish trust and reduce anxiety.
2. Speech therapy and cognitive behavioral therapy (CBT) to address underlying psychological factors.
3. Physical therapy or relaxation techniques for associated muscle tension or vocal strain.

Prognosis: With early diagnosis and appropriate intervention, FVSDs often show significant improvement. The approach emphasizes validation of symptoms, education, and collaborative care involving neurologists, psychiatrists, and speech therapists to optimize recovery.

Case example: A 65-year-old presenting with acute inability to speak but preserved comprehension may have a functional disorder, especially in the absence of other neurological deficits like hemiparesis or dysphagia. Initial workup should exclude stroke with imaging. Functional features such as variability, distractibility, and preserved automatic speech support diagnosis. Management follows the principles outlined above, emphasizing reassurance, therapy, and addressing psychological factors.

In contrast, a similar presentation in a child would probably not require ruling out stroke, as functional causes are more likely in younger patients without vascular risk factors.

CONCLUSION

FVSD can be reliably diagnosed through distinct patterns and positive signs, differentiating them from organic disorders. Early recognition and appropriate therapy lead to substantial recovery and improved quality of life.

Q29. Can one get functional urinary symptoms like inability to pass urine or frequency of micturition or feeling of incomplete evacuation?

Ans. Functional urinary symptoms are a recognized subset of functional disorders, diagnosed primarily through clinical history after excluding neurological, urological, or gynecological conditions.

Types of functional urinary symptoms are:
- *Storage dysfunction*: It includes urgency, increased frequency, nocturia, and urge incontinence.
- *Voiding dysfunction*: It involves urinary hesitancy, intermittent flow, slow stream, straining, incomplete bladder emptying, and urinary retention. Increased frequency and retention are particularly common.

Predisposing factors:
- Functional urinary retention is often observed in young females.
- Contributing factors include life stressors, unhappy family dynamics, or emotional deprivation during childhood. Some cases are linked to secondary gains, such as avoiding undesirable situations or reducing domestic responsibilities.

Associations: Functional urinary symptoms frequently occur alongside functional somatic syndromes (e.g., fibromyalgia, irritable bowel syndrome) or other functional neurological disorders, such as functional dystonia or weakness.

Management: Treatment focuses on:
- Identifying and addressing underlying psychological or emotional stressors
- Cognitive behavioral therapy (CBT)
- Pelvic floor exercises to improve voiding function and control

Proper diagnosis and sensitive management are essential for patient care. Let me know if you would like further clarification.

Q30. What are various functional neurological disorders (FNDs) in children? How they differ from FND in adults?

Ans. Functional neurological disorders are increasingly recognized in children, driven by factors such as academic pressure, family stress, and heightened exposure to social media. FND is more common in females and older children, with symptoms often linked to environmental and emotional stressors.

Common types of FNDs in children:

- *Functional motor symptoms*: These include weakness, movement disorders, and gait abnormalities. Children may show excessive effort or exaggerated postures while walking, which improve with distraction.
- *Functional seizures [psychogenic nonepileptic seizure (PNES)]*: PNES are prevalent in children, characterized by fluctuating symptoms, prolonged events, and inconsistent semiology such as asynchronous limb movements or side-to-side head movements.
- *Functional sensory symptoms*: These include visual loss, altered somatosensory perception, or unusual patterns of sensory deficits.
- *Other symptoms*: These include dizziness, abdominal pain, headache, frequent urination, and other somatic complaints which lack a clear organic basis.

Differences between children and adults:

- *Predisposing factors*: In children, common triggers include academic pressure, bullying, sibling rivalry, parental discord, or exposure to similar disorders in peers. Adults, on the other hand, frequently present with stressors related to relationships or financial pressures.
- *Symptom presentation*: Functional myoclonus and tics are more common in children, while facial movement disorders like functional hemifacial spasm are rare. The coronavirus disease 2019 (COVID-19) pandemic saw an increase in functional tic-like behaviors in children linked to social media exposure, such as the "TikTok tics" phenomenon.
- *Recovery rates*: Children typically experience higher rates of recovery compared to adults. Early diagnosis and intervention are pivotal to favorable outcomes.

Diagnosing FND in children: Key indicators include acute onset, fluctuating symptoms, inconsistencies between clinical findings and daily functioning, improvement with distraction, and the presence of identifiable stressors. For PNES, prolonged episodes with emotional manifestations (e.g., crying or grimacing) and preserved awareness can aid in differentiation from epileptic seizures.

Management: Effective management involves addressing underlying psychological and social factors through cognitive-behavioral therapy, family counseling, and physiotherapy. Educating families about the nature of FND is crucial to fostering cooperation and reducing stigma. With early and multidisciplinary care, children with FND often achieve significant recovery, underscoring the importance of timely intervention.

Q31. Clinical Scenarios: Recognizing and Managing Functional Neurological Disorder with Empathy and Comprehensive Care

SCENARIO 1: LEFT-SIDED WEAKNESS AND SENSORY DISTURBANCES

Patient presentation: Mrs PK, a 42-year-old woman, presents with a sudden onset of left-sided weakness and sensory disturbances in her left hand and leg. She is concerned about a potential stroke or brain disorder like tumor or need for brain surgery. She has no history of head injury.

Physician's Approach

History-taking:
Physician: "Mrs PK, thank you for coming in. I want to understand your symptoms fully. Can you describe when you first noticed the weakness and any events that preceded it?"

Mrs PK: "It started last week. I was at home, and suddenly, my left arm felt weak, and my leg felt numb. I went to the emergency department, and they did laboratory tests, electrocardiogram (ECG), and an magnetic resonance imaging (MRI) of my brain, which was normal. The doctor said there was nothing wrong, and it is just tension-related, but I still feel something is wrong. I'm worried that they have missed something."

Physician: "I understand your concern, Mrs PK. It must be very distressing to feel that something is wrong despite normal test results. Normal tests do not mean there's no problem. Let's explore this further. Have you experienced any injuries or illnesses around that time?"

Physical examination: The physician performs a detailed neurological examination, noting positive signs such as Hoover's sign, where weakness improves with contralateral movement.

Physician: "Mrs PK, I noticed that when you move your right leg, your left leg strength improves. This is a sign that can be seen in a condition called functional neurological disorder (FND). It doesn't mean you're faking symptoms; it's a real condition with multifaceted origins and presentations."

Diagnostic explanation:
Physician: "FND involves symptoms like weakness and sensory changes without structural damage seen on MRI. It doesn't require surgery and often improves with therapy. These symptoms are genuine and can be influenced by both neurological and psychological factors."

Mrs PK: "Does that mean my symptoms are all in my head?"

Physician: "Not at all. FND is a well-recognized condition involving how your brain processes movements and sensations. It's like a temporary problem in the brain's software, not hardware. It's reversible and treatable. We'll work together to improve it."

Treatment plan:
Physician: "I recommend a combination of physical therapy for weakness and counseling to address stress. This approach treats the whole person and is highly effective. We'll follow up weekly to monitor progress."

Mrs PK: "That sounds manageable. I want to get better. Thank you!"

SCENARIO 2: FUNCTIONAL TREMOR

Patient presentation: Mr AR, a 36-year-old man, reports a sudden onset of right-hand tremors that worsen during stress and improve when distracted.

Physician's Approach

History-taking:
Physician: "Mr AR, when did you first notice the tremor, and has anything specific triggered it?"

Mr AR: "About 3 weeks ago, after a big argument at work. It gets worse when I'm stressed."

Physician: "That's helpful information. Stress can sometimes affect how the brain regulates movement. Let's check further."

Physical examination: The physician performs entrainment testing and notes that the tremor reduces when Mr AR focuses on a different task.

Physician: "I noticed your tremor changes when you focus on your other hand. This is a feature we often see in functional neurological disorder, suggesting the movements are influenced by how your brain is processing signals, not structural damage."

Diagnostic explanation:
Physician: "This is called a functional tremor, and it's a real and treatable condition. It's like your brain is sending extra signals to the muscles. The good news is we can retrain the brain to stop this pattern."

Treatment plan:
Physician: "We'll start physiotherapy and distraction techniques, along with stress management strategies. Many people see significant improvement with this approach."

Mr AR: "That's reassuring. I'll give it a try."

SCENARIO 3: FUNCTIONAL SEIZURES

Patient presentation: Ms SD, a 29-year-old woman, presents with episodes of unresponsiveness and shaking that have no clear electroencephalogram (EEG) abnormalities.

Physician's Approach

History-taking:
Physician: "Can you describe what happens before, during, and after these episodes?"

Ms SD: "I feel anxious, my vision blurs, and then I lose control. Afterward, I feel exhausted."

Physical examination and observations:

- No postictal confusion.
- Normal EEG during an event

Diagnostic explanation:

Physician: "These episodes are called functional seizures. They are not epileptic, but they are real and caused by how the brain processes signals during stress. They respond well to therapy aimed at stress reduction and retraining responses."

Treatment plan:

Physician: "I recommend cognitive-behavioral therapy and grounding exercises to manage triggers. We'll review your progress regularly."

Ms SD: "That makes sense. I'm ready to start therapy."

CONCLUSION

These scenarios demonstrate compassionate, structured approaches to recognizing and managing FND. They emphasize clear explanations, validation, treatment plans addressing physical and emotional aspects, and establishing follow-up to build trust and encourage recovery.

SUGGESTED READINGS

For understanding the concept of functional neurological disorders:

1. Espay AJ, Aybek S, Carson A, et al. Current Concepts in Diagnosis and Treatment of Functional Neurological Disorders. JAMA Neurol. 2018;75(9):1132-41.
2. Bennett K, Diamond C, Hoeritzauer I, et al. A practical review of functional neurological disorder (FND) for the general physician. Clin Med (Lond). 2021;21(1):28-36.
3. Stone J, Carson A, Duncan R, et al. Which neurological diseases are most likely to be associated with "symptoms unexplained by organic disease". J Neurol. 2012;259(1):33-8.

Diagnostic pitfalls in functional neurological disorders:

1. Pimentel Filho LH, Mutarelli EG. Diagnostic pitfalls in functional neurological disorders. Arq Neuropsiquiatr. 2022;80(5 Suppl 1):324-7.
2. Finkelstein SA, Popkirov S. Functional Neurological Disorder: Diagnostic Pitfalls and Differential Diagnostic Considerations. Neurol Clin. 2023;41(4):665-79.

Implication of misdiagnosis of functional neurological disorders:

1. Baglioni V, Esposito D, Bernardi K, et al. Misdiagnosis of functional neurological symptom disorders in paediatrics: Narrative review and relevant case report. Clin Child Psychol Psychiatry. 2024;29(3):1026-42.
2. Mcloughlin C, Lee WH, Carson A, et al. Iatrogenic harm in functional neurological disorder. Brain. 2024:awae283.

Functional weakness and la belle indifference in functional neurological disorders:

1. Stone J, Aybek S. Functional limb weakness and paralysis. Handb Clin Neurol. 2016;139: 213-28.
2. Stone J, Smyth R, Carson A, et al. La belle indifférence in conversion symptoms and hysteria: Systematic review. Br J Psychiatry. 2006;188(3):204-9.
3. Tremolizzo L, Susani E, Riva MA, et al. Positive signs of functional weakness. J Neurol Sci. 2014;340(1-2):13-8.

Functional gait disorder:

1. Nonnekes J, Růžička E, Serranová T, et al. Functional gait disorders: A sign-based approach. Neurology. 2020;94(24):1093-9.
2. Edwards M. Functional (psychogenic) gait disorder: diagnosis and management. Handb Clin Neurol. 2018;159:417-23.

Psychogenic non epileptic seizures:

1. Deli A, Huang YG, Toynbee M, et al. Distinguishing psychogenic nonepileptic, mixed, and epileptic seizures using systemic measures and reported experiences. Epilepsy Behav. 2021;116:107684.
2. Dickinson P, Looper KJ. Psychogenic nonepileptic seizures: a current overview. Epilepsia. 2012;53(10):1679-89.

Functional movement disorders:

1. Park JE. Functional Movement Disorders: Updates and Clinical Overview. J Mov Disord. 2024;17(3):251-61.
2. Morgante F, Edwards MJ, Espay AJ. Psychogenic movement disorders. Continuum (Minneap Minn) 2013;19(5 Movement Disorders):1383-96.
3. Thenganatt MA, Jankovic J. Psychogenic tremor: a video guide to its distinguishing features. Tremor Other Hyperkinet Mov (N Y). 2014;4:253.
4. Akkaoui MA, Geoffroy PA, Roze E, et al. Functional Motor Symptoms in Parkinson's Disease and Functional Parkinsonism: A Systematic Review. J Neuropsychiatry Clin Neurosci. 2020 Winter;32(1):4-13.

Functional eye movement disorders:

1. Kaski D, Bronstein AM, Edwards MJ, et al. Cranial functional (psychogenic) movement disorders. Lancet Neurol. 2015;14(12):1196-205.
2. Kaski D, Bronstein AM. Functional eye movement disorders. Handb Clin Neurol. 2016;139:343-51.

Functional voice and speech disorders:

1. Baker J. Functional voice disorders: Clinical presentations and differential diagnosis. Handb Clin Neurol. 2016;139:389-405.
2. Duffy JR. Functional speech disorders: clinical manifestations, diagnosis, and management. Handb Clin Neurol. 2016;139:379-88.

Functional urological symptoms:

1. Hoeritzauer I, Phe V, Panicker JN. Urologic symptoms and functional neurologic disorders. Handb Clin Neurol. 2016:139:469-81.

Functional coma:

1. Ludwig L, McWhirter L, Williams S, et al. Functional coma. Handb Clin Neurol. 2016;139: 313-27.

Functional neurological disorders in children:

1. Yong K, Chin RFM, Shetty J, et al. Functional neurological disorder in children and young people: Incidence, clinical features, and prognosis. Dev Med Child Neurol. 2023;65(9): 1238-46.

Gender difference and risk factors in fucntional movement disorders:

1. Baizabal-Carvallo JF, Jankovic J. Gender Differences in Functional Movement Disorders. Mov Disord Clin Pract. 2019;7(2):182-7.
2. Fobian AD, Elliott L. A review of functional neurological symptom disorder etiology and the integrated etiological summary model. J Psychiatry Neurosci. 2019;44(1):8-18.

Understanding the pathophysiology of functional neurological disorders:

1. Drane DL, Fani N, Hallett M, et al. A framework for understanding the pathophysiology of functional neurological disorder. CNS Spectr. 2020:1-7.

2. Demartini B, Nisticò V, Edwards MJ, et al. The pathophysiology of functional movement disorders. Neurosci Biobehav Rev. 2021;120:387-400.

Management of functional neurological disorders:

1. Gilmour GS, Nielsen G, Teodoro T, et al. Management of functional neurological disorder. J Neurol. 2020;267(7):2164-72.
2. Baker J, Barnett C, Cavalli L, et al. Management of functional communication, swallowing, cough and related disorders: consensus recommendations for speech and language therapy. J Neurol Neurosurg Psychiatry. 2021;92:1112-25.

Index

Page numbers followed by *b* refer to box *f* refer to figure, *fc* refer to flowchart and *t* refer to table.

D

E

F

G

H

N

O